The Flexible Diet

Flexible dieting is the new buzzword in weight loss, and for good reason. Join the legions of people who are losing weight with ease, and eating foods they love while doing so. Discover the simple science behind weight loss, and how the freedom behind The Flexible Diet will make this book the last diet book you will ever need.

Discover how to;

Lose weight

Keep it off for life

Lose more fat

Retain more lean mass, so you look more defined

Feel fuller for longer

Eat foods you love while doing so

Do it all with minimal exercise

Free yourself from restrictive diets

The Flexible Diet

This book is designed to provide information that the author deems accurate on the subject matter at the time of writing. It is sold with the understanding that the author is offering no specific individualized advice, and holds no responsibility or liability for information implemented.

No warranty is made with the accuracy of the information contained within this book, nor the completeness. The author accepts no liability for loss, personal or otherwise, incurred as a consequence of the use and application of the information contained within this book.

This book presents the ideas of the Author, and is not meant to replace the qualified opinion of your professional healthcare practitioner. You must consult your professional healthcare practitioner before implementing any ideas within this book. The Author disclaims responsibility for any effects resulting directly or indirectly from implementing information from this book.

Copyright © 2015 by Adam Young

This book is Copyright

No reproduction without permission

All rights reserved

ISBN-13: 978-1519520456

ISBN-10: 151952045X

The right of Adam Young to be identified as the author of this work

www.TheFlexibleDiet.com

To my Parents – thank you for your constant love and support in all that I do.

To Lee – Thanks for all of your help

Table of Contents

INTRODUCTION - WHY ANOTHER DIET BOOK?	13
CHAPTER 1 - WHY DIETS WORK, AND WHY THEY FAIL	17
DIET PSYCHOLOGY	18
WHY DIETS FAIL	20
CHAPTER SUMMARY	25
CHAPTER 2 - ENERGY BALANCE	27
ENERGY STORAGE IN THE BODY	28
TIPPING THE BALANCE IN OUR FAVOUR	30
WHAT DO WE WANT FROM A DIET?	32
EAT WHAT YOU WANT – AND LOSE WEIGHT	32
SCIENTIFIC PROOF	39
WOULD WE EVER WANT TO LIMIT INSULIN?	43
NAIL IN THE COFFIN	45
SUGGESTIONS AND LESSONS	45
BREAKFAST AND METABOLISM	47
MEAL SIZE AND FREQUENCY REGARDING WEIGHT GAIN	51
FINAL THOUGHTS	54
CHAPTER SUMMARY	55
SECTION 2 - THE DIET	57
CHAPTER 3 - CRON	59
WHAT CAN WE DO ABOUT THIS?	60
BENEFITS OF CRON	61
LONG TERM BENEFITS OF CRON	62
WHY CRON WORKS	63

How to Do It	64
Chapter Summary	74

CHAPTER 4 - CALORIE CYCLING / DISTRIBUTION — 75

What is Calorie Cycling/Distribution?	75
Alternate Day	78
Psychological Benefits	82
How to Do It	83
Chapter Summary	86

CHAPTER 5 - MACROS, MICROS AND FOOD CHOICES — 87

Carbohydrates	87
Fats	89
Protein – the Magic Macro	91
Micros	95
How to Do It	97
Examples	101
Chapter Summary	104

CHAPTER 6 - EXERCISE — 105

Types of Training	109
How to Do It	113
The Program	120
Calories	124
Chapter Summary	128

CHAPTER 7 - WHEN SHOULD I EAT? — 129

Meal Frequency	129
Meal Skipping	134
Nutrient Timing	140

CHAPTER SUMMARY	146

CHAPTER 8 - WHEN NOT TO EAT — 147
WHO FASTS?	148
WHAT HAPPENS WHEN WE FAST?	148
METABOLIC RATE	149
FASTING IS DIFFICULT	150
FASTING AND WEIGHT LOSS	150
BENEFITS TO HEALTH	152
TYPES OF FASTING	154
NOT SO FAST	157
NUTRIENT TIMING AND FASTING	158
FLEXIBILITY	161
CHAPTER SUMMARY	162

CHAPTER 9 - EXAMPLES — 163
SAMPLE DAYS	163
WEEKLY PLANS	167

CHAPTER 10 - FLEXIBILITY — 173
FITTING IT INTO YOUR LIFE	175
THE MAINTENANCE DAY	178
FLEXIBILITY WITH MACROS AND MICROS	179

SECTION 3 - MENTAL — 183
INTRODUCTION TO MENTAL — 185

CHAPTER 11 - GOAL SETTING 187
- EXCITE YOURSELF 188
- DREAM BIG, BUT NOT TOO BIG 190
- LONG TERM/SHORT TERM 191
- CHAPTER SUMMARY 195

CHAPTER 12 - MOTIVATION 197
- THE WHY 198
- USING NEGATIVES 201
- VISION BOARD 205
- THE SUCCESS BOARD 206
- SOCIAL ACCOUNTABILITY 208
- THE MORNING RITUAL 210
- OVERCOMING OBSTACLES 212
- CHAPTER SUMMARY 214

CHAPTER 13 - PLANNING AND PERIODIZATION 215
- PERIODIZATION AND BREAKS 216
- PLANNING 220
- ASSESSMENT AND EVALUATION 223
- RE-EVALUATING 233

CHAPTER 14 - END NOTES 239
- MAINTENANCE OF THE 'NEW YOU' 240

BOOK SUMMARY 243
REFERENCES 247

The Flexible Diet

Eat the foods you love, lose the weight you hate

Introduction - Why Another Diet Book?

Why another diet book? Don't we have enough already? Why do we have such an obesity epidemic when we have all this information out there to help us? Does any of it work?

There are a plethora of diet books on the market right now. Most of them prey on the hope of others, with claims of unsustainable and unrealistic amounts of weight loss. Almost all of them prescribe very specific rules which, if you veer away from, you are doomed for failure. Most require cutting out all your favourite foods and eating nothing but the set menu they provide for you, leaving you longing and craving for those tasty meals you once had when life was fun.

You get to the point where you are losing weight simply from the fact you recoil in horror at having to wolf down another 'low carb, low fat, low everything' dish. You dread those social functions where you may have to eat something that doesn't comply with your strict regimen, thus spoiling all your efforts from previous weeks. Hardly motivating, right?

What if there was a diet that you could make your own; one that didn't require cutting out all your favourite foods? One that is not so strict and also gives you the long term success and freedom you desire. A more sensible and realistic approach to dieting that allows you to still eat what you want and lose weight, and is backed by science. One that not only makes you lose weight, but actually more of it from your fat stores, resulting in a leaner and more toned look as well as the desired numbers on the scales. What if there was a diet that could make you enjoy the process a little more; even enjoy it fully? Even enjoy it so much that you prefer dieting! Surely not? A diet that still allows the good things in life; the foods that taste really good which are supposed to be so bad for you. These are pretty wild claims in themselves, but they become much more possible when you follow The Flexible Diet.

This book explores the reasons behind every diet that works and every diet that doesn't. In reading this you will understand the underlying mechanisms of every successful diet, allowing you to formulate a plan which follows the best advice and negates the worst. Unfortunately, there is a lot of poor information out there amongst all the magazine articles, books, newspaper columns and online forums. But, within each, there are elements of truth, masked by a veil of misunderstanding, misinterpretation or plain lies.

The world is a scary place right now, with carbohydrates, sugar, fats and even protein all being hailed as the cause of our obesity epidemic. If we listened to all the nonsense in the media, there would be nothing left for us to eat anymore. But losing weight doesn't have to be a minefield of confusion. Through understanding and applying the principles of The Flexible Diet, you will be well on your way to lifelong weight management, while still being able to enjoy your food (even more so than before).

Through correct knowledge you can become 'diet enlightened', allowing you to take control of your own destiny and enabling you with the real truths that allow you to be shielded from the day to day rubbish that gets thrown around. Will this book explain those truths – yes. It will also use scientific information to correctly back up any claims. At the back of this book you will also find all of those sources noted so that you can check them yourselves and be sure of their interpretations.

Maybe you are obese, maybe not. Maybe you are just looking to lose a little winter weight in time for the beach season. Perhaps you have a wedding coming up, a holiday or some event where you would like to look a little more in shape. Maybe you would like to lose weight for health reasons or perhaps you just want to feel good about your everyday appearance and would like to achieve that goal in a sensible and realistic way. This book will free you from the shackles of every other diet and allow you to create a way of living which suits you. One that is flexible, and one that you are allowed to (even encouraged to) periodically relax from.

Everyone has a different lifestyle, and you need a diet that suits yours or it simply will not work. Some people are not able to follow plans where you eat every 2 hours (this myth will be debunked in good time anyway) and some people can't handle eating little or no carbohydrates each day (again this will be cast out). A diet that works is one that works with and for you, not against you.

This book will take you through a journey of understanding, explaining dieting myths, why diets work and why they don't. Then comes the fun part, the instructional keys to successful dieting are explained in 'The Flexible Diet' section. This section will cover the main keys to weight loss, and will also explain how to keep the weight falling off consistently over a longer period of time. Also explained in this section of the book are ways to improve *fat* loss specifically (as opposed to just pure weight loss). This is what we really want when we are talking about weight loss.

When we lose fat, we end up with a slender more toned physique that fits into clothes better, and we are able to maintain that fat loss for longer. Dieting usually causes people to lose too much lean body mass rather than fat, and this is not good for your long term weight loss. A lot of diets are rather unhealthy in terms of cutting out certain things, leading to less variation in food choices; not so with this diet. The other keys in this section will show you how to maintain a healthy lifestyle while continuing with your weight loss goals, and keep your body functioning optimally. Also discussed are the areas of exercising your body; essential parts in long term weight loss and maintenance of a lean physique. We look at the realities of exercise, and find a plan which can fit into what you can do, which could be as little as 20 minutes, 3 times a week.

This book also includes basic psychological tools that will enable you to maximize your adherence to your goals, and achieve them in a more positive and constructive way, making you feel like every day is a step forward. Diet books have a tendency to forget most of these important elements and hence adherence is normally very low; if not for the diet itself being insanely difficult to maintain, but the lack of psychological control allowing those demons to come back in to play.

This diet is not a strict formula, but a series of important keys and tools. You needn't do all of the key elements, but the more motivated you are and the more keys you utilize, the better your results will be. You can read through some of the chapters and decide if the idea presented is right for you, if it fits with you and your life. If you think it will be easy to implement, then go ahead. If not, then you can leave it until a later date to bring in, or leave it completely.

However, it should be noted that all elements of this diet can be completely natural to you once practiced and ingrained in your life. Just like any skill, at first it may seem difficult or even impossible, but with practice it becomes easier and easier until you no longer even have to think about it. I would recommend trying all of the pieces of this diet at least once, as you may find it is the major factor in you achieving success much faster and easier.

The Flexible Diet takes the approach of long term success. Part of this is achieved through the knowledge presented (knowledge is power), so I would recommend reading through all the sections of the book. However, if you are really impatient, you can skip straight to the diet section. The format of the book makes it easy to dip in and out of, so that once you have read it and understood it you can use it as a reference any time your weight loss journey gets stagnant or needs re-energizing.

There are summaries at the end of each section; these will act as reminders for you after you have read all of the information. Rather than having to re-read the book, you can simply turn to the summary sections and have all of the chapters' information re-called. Good luck with your path to a new you, enjoy every moment of it.

Chapter 1

Why Diets Work, And Why They Fail

This chapter will explore in more detail why some diets work and why others don't, leaving us with lessons to take and apply to ourselves.

You will start to get an idea for where the diet section of this book will go, and by educating yourself in the following ideas you can become your own nutritionist. People are always looking for advice or information telling them exactly what to do in the hope that they will stumble across a simple secret to weight loss. People never really learn to take ownership of that knowledge, and hence have no long term control. But this information often has some short term success. Why do these diets have success? Maybe if we can see what makes them tick we could use that principle, and dust off the rest of the rubbish.

Most diets sell on a hook, some kind of 'magic bullet' that is supposed to work for you, such as eating foods from a limited list, avoiding food combining (another bizarre concept I won't even attempt to waste paper on), cutting carbs, cutting fats, cutting foods with any vowels in their names etc. While these are all ridiculous and completely unnecessary ideas, they still work for the most part (especially short term).

The physiological reasons for their success are simple; by eliminating certain foods through the above methods, you are finding a no-brain way of cutting calories. Whether a diet uses a points system, a set meal plan, or use of specific foods that are more satiating, they are all basically ways of making you eat less energy.

If someone told you that in order to lose weight you must limit carbohydrates to less than 20 grams per day in your diet (this is the typical protocol for Low – Carb), it doesn't really leave you with many food options. For a start, most foods have a certain carbohydrate value, so allowing only 20 grams per day will force you to eat less overall. Also, by eliminating carbohydrates, people are forced to eat higher fat and higher protein foods, which tend to keep you fuller for longer. On the other end of the scale, a diet that is low in fat will act in a more direct calorie control way. It is not that cutting fat makes you lose weight, but by eliminating this nutrient you are taking away a source of high calories. However, we see that this eventually fails, as people end up over-consuming other foods to make up for the loss of fat in their diet.

Diet Psychology

The psychological reasons for the success of diets are also straightforward. For the most part, people reach a low point in their lives where they are simply not happy with themselves. Although we tend to view these low points as negative, they actually serve a purpose for us in drastically improving our motivation to change for the better. As a 'contented person', you are far less likely to make positive changes to further improve yourself. In fact, we will take control of this mechanism later on in the book and use it to our advantage. When people get to a low point in their lives and decide to make the change, they will tend to seek out information, of which there is plentiful supply in this great age of technology.

If you believe in anything strongly enough, you will make it work. If the idea of the magic bullet being proposed is logical to you and is sold in the correct way (hyped up sensationalism and pseudo-scientific claims often are the order of the day), then we become convinced of its effectiveness. Often, we will even tell others about the diet (if we are convinced enough that it will work). This gives us something called social accountability. By the diet being hyped up to us, we subsequently hype it up further to others in an attempt to make it sound more interesting and astounding than it already seemed when you were first introduced to the idea. If the book proposes potential weight losses of 5 pounds a week, we often tell others claims of 10 pound per week are not uncommon (come on,

I'll bet you've been guilty of this). As you get glares of intrigue (or rather disbelief) from your fellow workers about your claims, it switches a trigger in our brains to prove ourselves right (or prove their scepticism wrong). As a result, your compliance to the diet increases dramatically; after all, we wouldn't want to look stupid now, would we?

This psychological phenomenon is often used to great effect by magicians who find that most of the 'magic' is done after the trick by people exaggerating the event in their mind and to others. The story of an amazing magic trick can very quickly become more and more elaborate with each telling until the trick no longer resembles the original. But this observable fact doesn't just happen in magic, just listen to any child re-telling stories of what happened after a particular event. We never seem to get rid of this ability to exaggerate even as we get older (how big was the fish you caught?).

Social accountability is not the only psychological phenomenon helping diets work. While it is a good form of external motivation, there is a great deal of internal accountability. The act of dieting or saying to oneself, "I am going on a diet", has several implications for how we conduct ourselves day to day. When you are in 'dieting mode', you instantly become more aware of your food choices and portion sizes. Maybe you even add in an exercise regimen to speed up your rate of success. We are less inclined to over-eat, or over-indulge, and our minds instantly seek out healthier alternatives - we all know deep down how to lose weight.

These healthier alternatives are often more satiating and induce less addictive eating behaviours, serving us in lowering our overall daily energy intake. Our mind-set also changes from a state of feeling 'rewarded' for eating tasty food and stuffing ourselves, to the opposite - 'guilt' for over eating or eating the wrong foods. In a synergistic fashion, our attitude changes to a 'rewarded feeling' towards better food choices and a 'guilty feeling' when these foods lack in our diet.

Most of this would fall under the category of 'Hawthorne effect', where the simple act of increased awareness can spark a change in behaviour. This was first demonstrated in 1924, when workers were studied to see which type of lighting (brighter or dimmer) produced highest work efficiencies. To their surprise, both the dimmer and the brighter lights increased work-rate; the simple act of being aware of the study produced a response in the workers similar to that of a dieter being more aware of food choices.

We also love seeing the numbers fly off the scales in the honeymoon period. And while our attention is directed towards this, it becomes a great source of motivation, further improving our adherence to the diet. But all physiological and psychological ideas aside, there are no magic bullets. When you search for the common denominators in the diets circulated since dieting has begun, they all point to one thing as being the reason for their success – an idea which is the central premise of this book.

Why Diets Fail

The history of dieting hasn't been very good; short term successes have often been counterbalanced by long term failures. Or even worse - when people gain back more weight than they originally lose. Society wants a quick fix, and there are fast routes to almost everything these days. Faster cars, faster computers, faster information, and if we can't have it now we just look for someone or something that tells us we can. But quicker is not always better.

Gaining fat was actually a good survival strategy for humans when we were strolling the plains of Africa. Only very recently has food been in plentiful supply; unfortunately, it is not equally distributed over the world. Gaining fat through eating energy dense foods is genetically encoded in each of us. During times of famine, these fat stores would then be used to fuel our metabolism and allow us to continue until the next feast came along. Unfortunately, our current comfortable situations prevent famine from ever happening to us in the developed world. When you are hungry, there are a whole host of delicious options to satiate your every desire. And without natural famine to counterbalance that fact, we have to often induce our own in the form of dieting (or not at all in the case of obesity).

As a result of our evolutionary desire to consume energy dense foods, we have gotten ourselves into quite a mess. Obesity epidemics are rising rapidly along with the diseases they bring. And while dieting goes against our genetic makeup (it is not of an evolutionary advantage to get pleasure out of losing weight), the correct answer would be to try to keep our body in a more level state regarding weight. However, the majority of people reading this book are already overweight, so we need a method to put ourselves in that uncomfortable anti-evolutionary position called dieting, but make it as comfortable as possible through the process. This book is the answer to that. So why are other diets failing in the long term?

We Are Not Designed to Lose Weight

The first answer is given above; basically our body does not want to lose weight. When we try, our body fights us in an attempt to keep our fat levels high. Fat reserves give us an advantage in the wild over someone without; but we are no longer in the wild, and the advantage it used to serve is now meaningless. But this 'fight' that our body gives remains with us to this day.

Levels of the hormone 'Leptin' drop, Ghrelin and Cortisol increase, escalating the hunger levels which make us hate dieting. While motivation is high, this is normally not a problem. But how long can you spend in a hungry state before you give up? This is one of the major reasons behind most diet failures and will be addressed in The Flexible Diet.

Our body also responds to lower food intakes by eventually slowing our metabolism down to match how much food is coming in, thus decreasing the effect of the diet over time. While this is largely unavoidable, there are certain tactics that The Flexible Diet will employ to counter the metabolic drop.

Limited food choices of current diets also induce other physiologically undesirable effects. By lacking flexibility and variability we are not providing the best for our health. Variability in the diet is very important, as almost all forms of food offer benefits, whether through different types of vitamins and minerals or different micro-compositions that our body needs. When lacking in these varying vitamins/minerals and micro-compositions (for example, different types of meat contain different amino acid profiles, and consuming a variety of sources can be very beneficial), our body can sense the deficit and responds with either feelings of sluggishness or energy loss and/or a compromised immune system, often leading to illnesses.

This often happens when carbohydrates or fats are taken out of the diet for example. 'Low carbers' will tend to suffer carb crashing, which is similar to a marathon runner hitting the wall at the 20 hour mark. Although this is only temporary as our bodies switch over to ketosis (a different way of fuelling itself), often it is too much for people to handle, and the long term effects of staying in this state have not been researched enough.

The long term undesirable physiological effects of most diets are also numerous, with one of the main ones being muscle loss. Most diets are not set up in a way that promotes retention of muscle, and long term dieting will tend to leave you with much lower levels of lean body mass after it. This will prove a great disservice to you in your goal to look lean, toned and young. It also will dramatically reduce your ability to maintain your new low weight, as retention of lean body mass helps us to keep the weight off for good (through various mechanisms).

Although muscle loss is an almost unavoidable effect of dieting, The Flexible Diet will go through specific strategies to minimize this and possibly increase levels for some. I am not talking about waking up and looking like a bodybuilder one day, but just maintaining enough so that your physique looks much more slender, toned and shapely.

Motivation

Most diets are simply not set up in a way that promotes motivation and/or willpower. Their content (choice), structure and lack of motivational tools mean that people can only stay on the diet for so long before they lose their will and discontinue. Here is the kicker - and most of you will have experienced this before if you have ever been on a diet - when you stop the diet, often you will respond with a gorge of all the foods that have been forbidden.

In the case of low carbohydrate diets, we are obviously going to respond by consumption of excess sugary delights, tingling our taste buds with every mouthful and setting off a chain reaction of more and more until….. all of the glycogen stores we depleted during our low carb phase become replete (and then some) along with all the water we lost in that first heavenly week. Cue big weight gain, depression, followed by comfort eating, followed by more weight gain and so forth in a vicious cycle until we come to the conclusion that diets simply don't work, at least until the next one comes along with enough hype to make us try it.

A lack of choice eventually gets to us for a very 'human' reason; when we are forbidden anything, whether a food or activity, most of us instinctively want to do that thing even more. A study with kids showed just how instinctive this is, as they were told they could play with any toy in the room apart from 'that one'. When the adults left the room and monitored the children remotely, it's not difficult to imagine what they saw – the kids went straight for the outlawed toy.

The same idea applies to adults (sometimes even more so), and especially dieting. A carbohydrate free diet may be ecstatically pleasing initially, as people fry eggs, bacon, sausages and wolf them down cackling to themselves at the delight of how they've won the dieting lottery, able to lose weight by eating these foods. But two weeks later, these same people are sick to death of the lack or variability, reminiscing about the days where they ate a slice of bread without fear, or enjoyed a chocolate bar, letting the sugary sweetness melt in their mouth and envelop their taste buds in a sea of smooth, creamy delight (is your mouth watering yet?). By the fourth week, when the initial water loss has stopped and weight loss severely slows down, they begin to question the benefits of the diet when weighed against their ever increasing desire to gobble a box of doughnuts. Cue diet failure. Although the above example has been directed more towards a low carb diet, the same applies to a diet cutting out any foods with the letter 'A' in it (I don't know if this diet exists but I'm sure it would have the same effects).

The take home lessons are obvious, and the answers simple. Don't cut out foods, just find a way of using them sensibly in your dieting so that your weight loss is sustainable for longer and you don't get those yearnings that eventually sabotage your own success. Variety is also key for health and psychological longevity, so we definitely do not want to minimize choice.

All diets work, and they all work on one principle – energy balance. However, this is also the reason why all diets eventually fail, apart from The Flexible Diet. We must have ways around this point of failure so we can go through it without our success ever stopping. We must also realize that our psychology is as important as the diet itself.

The Flexible Diet will supply you with the much needed motivational tools (both psychological and physiological) to get through any problems you have with the minimum of fuss. A diet by nature is something you couldn't stick to long term. I hate to use the cliché term thrown about by every other diet, but this must be a lifestyle change (although an easy one to implement). It may not give the fastest results, but a diet that is easy to stick to, suits your lifestyle, allows you to eat all the types of food you want and motivates you every step of the way is the one that you will continue for life, and over the long term is the diet that you will see the best and longest lasting results with.

The boredom factor of most diets is very apparent to anyone who has ever been on one. Not with The Flexible Diet. In fact, it opens up so many more options to you than ever before that it can make your diet more variable than your old ways of eating. This is The Flexible Diet. So what are we waiting for, let's get started.

Chapter Summary

Often, negative emotion is the fuel which sparks a dramatic weight loss

Social accountability massively improves our ability to lose weight

Diets work because they create an energy deficit – less energy is coming in than going out

This is usually achieved by creating a restriction in choice, which indirectly creates an energy deficit

This lack of choice is ultimately what makes a diet fail, as when we cut out food groups/choices, we subconsciously desire them

We are not designed to lose weight – our body fights it through a cascade of hormonal changes designed to make you lose motivation.

While motivation is high in the early stages of dieting, we can deal with a lot of the negative elements. But ultimately, we realize that we cannot stay living that way, and so we come off the diet (hard).

Variety is healthy both physically and mentally – and will aid you in creating a diet you can adhere to

The Flexible diet will overcome these issues, and also use them to our advantage to improve adherence and enjoyment of the dieting process

Chapter 2
Energy Balance

This is the real key to weight loss, and the major theme of this book. In order to lose weight, you simply have to find a way of tipping the energy balance in your favour. What does this mean exactly?

Energy balance consists of two simple elements - energy in and energy out. If energy coming into your body is less than energy going out, we will lose weight. A simple analogy would be your bank account. Money is going out all the time and coming in all the time (hopefully). Depending on what the ratios are between the two, you can end the day with more or less money than you started. If you burned (or spent) 2000 calories (dollars) in a day and only ate (deposited) 1500 calories (dollars), then your body's energy stores (bank account) will be 500 calories in debt, equalling weight loss and probably a letter from your bank manager. Take this same analogy and apply it over the term of a month and we can have greater amounts of calorie debt and hence energy loss from our body.

It is quite 'in Vogue' at the moment to state the idea that energy balance is irrelevant for weight loss; there seems to be a backlash against the whole thermodynamics theory. However, it is important to remember that

No one has ever gained weight while in a calorie deficit. And EVERY clinically controlled trial with reduced calories shows weight loss, regardless of the type of food eaten.

I am talking here, of course, about true weight loss. Water levels fluctuate from day to day and can account for most of the rapid weight gains and losses you see in short periods of time; This is a very important concept to understand. When you step on the scales the night after a big meal only to see you have gained 4 pounds, it is practically impossible that you acquired 4 pounds of solid fat (unless your meal was over 14,000 calories). The very likely candidate is that your body is simply storing excess water.

This is the reason why most people who come off a diet can gain a lot of weight back in a short period of time; they are basically re-hydrating themselves. An extreme example of this is seen in the sport of bodybuilding. While preparing for a competition (especially in the last few days), the athletes will dehydrate themselves via cutting carbohydrates, varying their sodium levels and other tactics such as alcohol consumption. This serves the purpose of flushing their body of water, which is obviously not a very healthy state to remain in for too long. This allows a bodybuilder to walk on stage with very thin skin, allowing every striation in their muscles to be on full show. But this is what I would deem 'fake' weight loss.

To highlight this, after a competition has finished, a bodybuilder can easily put on upwards of 15 pounds in weight over the course of a day – almost all of it water. Unfortunately, this water flushing trick is one of the main secrets behind the short term success of a low carbohydrate diet. It is also why these diets fail so miserably when people stop this diet. People put back on all the water they lost during the initial weeks – which then makes them scared of carbohydrates even further.

This trick is also used by boxers trying to 'make-weight'. During the weigh in, they will be so dehydrated that they will actually be very weak. When you watch them in the actual fight, they are far more 'plump' as they have put on all the water they lost for the weigh in.

Energy Storage in the Body

If your body is overweight, it is simply storing more energy than you would like. This may have been built up over a shorter period of time through binge eating, or more commonly through a prolonged period of unnoticeable calorie excess. Prepare yourself now as we are about to get a little 'Sciency'. I promise to try to keep this as brief as possible.

The human body stores energy in three main forms;

Muscle

Glycogen

Fat

Our body has a certain lean mass, which consists of muscle, bone and organs amongst other things. For the most part, this is relatively static and genetically determined. In terms of storage, our body can hold energy in the form of muscle which can be broken down if necessary to provide energy. Some people naturally hold a lot of muscle on their body, while others are stick thin in terms of muscle mass. While most of this is genetically determined, people can increase the ability of their body to store energy as muscle through exercise and diet manipulations (or drugs, but we won't go into these here).

Muscle, or lean body mass, is also affected by a multitude of hormones which differ between genders and age groups. Generally, females have lower levels of the hormones which build and maintain muscle, while men have higher levels; in both sexes this tends to decline with aging. It is generally very difficult for our body to store energy as muscle. It is usually not of an evolutionary advantage, as muscle is much more difficult to convert into energy should we need it. Also, muscle tends to use more energy, which was a great disadvantage 10,000 years or so ago when food was scarce. This means that our body will naturally resist storing energy in this form, unless there is some external stimulus telling our body that it needs bigger and stronger muscles (coming in the form of weight training, usually). The stimulus is not the only thing needed to build muscle - we must have an excess of food so that our body feels there is enough energy around that it can safely undertake this job. That is why bodybuilders eat so much and fatten up during muscle building phases.

The body can also store a limited amount of energy in the form of glycogen (stored sugar), which can readily be converted into blood sugar and used throughout the day. The body can store glycogen in muscle, liver and other cells in the body. It is commonly accepted that for every gram of glycogen stored in the body there is another 3-4 grams of water stored with it (Kreitzman et al, 1992). With the amount of glycogen that can be stored in the body, it means that theoretically as much as 5 Kilograms or 11.25 pounds of weight can be lost without any fat loss whatsoever. This is the 'water weight' that we were discussing earlier. Muscle glycogen is used to power muscular movement for day to day purposes, or also during exercise. Liver glycogen is used to fuel the rest of the cells in the body.

Lastly, we have fat. We wished we didn't, but we do, and it is actually very healthy to have a certain amount of fat on our body. The problem comes when we store it in excess, creating difficulties in our health and other situations that we would prefer not deal with. If you are reading this book (which you are) then it is probable that you have an excess of this energy store and are looking to have less of it. Fat stores are built up when we have excess energy coming in. If that excess energy is not being used to build muscle, and our glycogen stores are already full, then fat storage ensues. While it is not as 'black and white' as this, it is a useful enough description to explain how fat gain happens.

Tipping the Balance in Our Favour

Our body is in a constant state of flux; energy is coming in and going out at all times. We are literally being built up and broken down at the same time. This is known as anabolism (building up) and catabolism (breaking down). What matters most is the balance between the two at the end of the hour, day, week, month and year.

While we would not necessarily notice changes from hour to hour, weekly fluctuations or longer are very detectable. Changes in our weight are a result of accumulations of small changes that are built up over time. An extra 500 calories being stored in your body will be completely unnoticeable, but continue this every day and you can gain up to 50 pounds of weight in a year.

We can tip the balance of energy in our body in two ways - changing energy coming in or energy going out. If we have more energy coming in than is going out we are going to gain energy; this is simple mathematics (and physics), and has been demonstrated in enough scientific studies to be irrefutable. As stated earlier, this energy can be stored in muscle, glycogen or fat. This is dependent upon many things; what form that energy comes in, your genetics, what your hormones are doing, if you have exercised or not and many other variables. This is what causes weight gain.

It is not a simple case of all the excess energy being shuttled into one area. Your body does not just decide to put all excess energy into your fat stores sometimes, or replenish glycogen stores on other occasions. It is a varying process, with nutrients being stored in different places on a continuum. Usually, the more depleted you are in one form of energy store, the quicker that gets replenished. If your stores of glycogen are rock bottom, usually they will get replenished before fat stores, although storage of both fat and glycogen will happen at the same time only in differing percentages. The total amount of energy stored in the body is still the same, but the place in which the energy is stored can be different. This is called energy or nutrient partitioning.

The reverse is true; if we have more energy going out than coming into our body, we will lose energy. This energy must come from breaking the body down, utilizing stored forms of glycogen, muscle tissue and, more preferably, fat stores. When your body is in a catabolic state, it can draw energy out from all three sources. We could break down muscle and convert that into sugars which can be used for energy, or we could use the glycogen stored in our liver. Also, the body could choose to burn fat, converting this into energy that can be used by the cells. All three of these are happening simultaneously at any one time in the body; depending on the ratios of each, energy can be lost from one source more predominantly than the other. But regardless of where that energy comes from, if your body has less energy coming in than going out, you will lose energy and consequently weight.

So What Do We Want from A Diet?

The perfect scenario for us would be to place our body in an energy deficit, where less energy is coming in than is being burned. Our body would start to utilize its own stores of energy, thus making us lose energy and weight. Ideally, all of this energy would come from fat stores, leaving our muscle stores untouched. Although genetics have a large role in where our body draws the energy from, we have a big influence on it through the tactics suggested in this book. Regardless of genetics, the suggestions in this diet will promote the best partitioning of that energy in terms of both how it goes into your body and how it comes out.

However, we have seen from our information on 'why diets fail' that there are numerous obstacles to overcome. The biggest problem by far is the fact that our body does not want to be in this state of deprivation. Whether this deprivation comes in the form of cutting out certain foods or nutrients, or simply from calorie restriction itself, our body will resist. So we need numerous tactics to make this process as easy and unnoticeable as possible. The strategies presented in this book will not only achieve that, but they can actually make dieting enjoyable. This will allow you to sustain the diet for longer, perhaps indefinitely, resulting in maximum control of your weight with minimum amount of hassle.

Eat What You Want – And Lose Weight

While this title sounds too good to be true, it will become a reality for you. One of the defining things about The Flexible Diet, and the element that makes it different from every other diet, is the fact that you can eat all your favourite foods with absolutely no restrictions. Read that last line again and make sure it has sunk in.

Yes, you can literally eat any food you want during this diet. Using the strategies presented in the next few chapters, you can still lose weight and make sure that most of it is coming from fat. This is exciting stuff. No longer do you have to cut out your treats, eating nothing but bland set-menus, or the same foods over and over again. If you want to eat cake, go ahead. If you want to eat ice cream, cream buns, chocolate, then be my guest. Am I advocating you stuff your face silly with nothing but treats? Of course not, but you need to make this diet your own by including foods that work well with your lifestyle, allergies, budget and of course, your taste-buds. You need to live life and enjoy food.

How can this be? Surely a diet that allows me to eat what I want is the same diet I am already on, which is obviously not working. Well, yes and no. The diet you are on currently is not working because of the energy balance that we talked about. The same diet that is failing you currently can be used to great effect if you find a way of tipping the balance of energy in your favour. And that is what the tactics of this book describe. You can still enjoy all the foods you currently do, as long as you obey the energy balance rule. That last sentence sums it up completely. You must get your energy balance correct and it must be enjoyable.

While this book is not going to tell you what to eat, it will offer you suggestions on foods that can help you in achieving your goal. Certain foods will help you with partitioning for example, increasing the amount of energy lost from fat stores and decreasing the amount of energy lost from muscle stores. We also want to try to create a diet that allows optimal health to develop. Again, suggestions will be made to help these causes. But it would go against the whole concept of the book to force you into a defined meal plan, as it would no longer be flexible and 'yours'.

I'm sure there are many questions that you have, hopefully they will be fully answered through the course of this book. But here are a couple of common things people have to say regarding the 'eat what you want' philosophy.

I've heard that eating fat causes you to be fat. Shouldn't I cut fat out of my diet?

The argument here is that dietary fat is stored in our body more easily than carbohydrates or protein. While this is true (it is very easy for your body to store dietary fat as body fat), it is not very wise to follow the strategy of cutting dietary fat. Apart from being extremely unhealthy, cutting fat out of your diet will not create weight loss unless there is an overall energy deficit in your diet. Conversely, eating fat does not cause you to get fat unless there is an energy increase above what you expend during the day. Fat does contain a lot of calories (9 calories per gram compared to 4 calories for carbohydrates and protein), so cutting out dietary fat is an efficient way to reduce the amount of calories coming in. However, Fat is also needed by our body for hormonal balance, vitamin absorption, metabolic rate and many other processes that are important to health.

We have to think of the bigger picture as always. Your body needs a certain amount of energy per day, usually referred to as your TDEE or total daily energy expenditure. This includes energy needed by cells in your body for normal functioning as well as day to day activity levels and any exercise you do. This energy will either be burned from the food we eat, or if we don't have enough energy in our blood at the time we will break down our energy stores. It's similar to using your bank savings when you don't have enough cash on you.

So even if you ate a very fatty meal, maybe 1000 calories of pure fat, you would still lose fat at the end of the day if you had burned 2000 calories through the day with your TDEE. You eat 1000 calories of fat, perhaps 200 calories go towards your metabolism and the other 800 calories of fat gets stored. But your TDEE is still ticking through the day; it still needs another 1800 calories. If that entire TDEE requirement comes from fat, then you end up losing 1000 calories of fat at the end of the day.

This analogy is the same whether you ingest a similar amount of carbohydrates protein or fat, with subtle differences in what is called the thermic effect of food; this is energy lost through breaking down and converting the food into something more useful.

But we will discuss this a little later on. The same idea is used for carbohydrates, a nutrient that people are increasingly (but unnecessarily) afraid of. If you were to ingest 1000 calories of carbohydrates, some would go towards your metabolism and some would be stored. But if you are in a negative energy balance at the end of the day, it doesn't matter; whatever you stored will be burned away later to fuel your TDEE needs. Saying that eating 1000 calories of fat or 1000 calories of carbohydrates is going to make you gain weight is as logical as saying "Putting money into your bank account makes you a richer person". While from the outside it makes sense, if you are spending more money than you are putting in, you're not going to be getting rich fast.

I've heard Carbohydrates are bad as they spike your insulin and hence make you fat?

There is a very common and annoying myth that is being perpetuated endlessly, especially in recent years with the rise of the glycemic index and low carb dieting. The myth goes like this;

"Eating carbohydrates forces your body to release insulin. Insulin is the hormone that helps you store fat and prevents your body from burning fat. Therefore, eating carbohydrates makes you fatter".

It is so tempting to believe this myth as it sounds so logical, and even nutritionists and health magazines are jumping on the bandwagon of this one before thinking it through. But it is flawed on so many levels.

While it is true that insulin has a role in storing fat and inhibiting breakdown of fat, it is not the only role. It also helps convert sugar in the blood into glycogen to be stored in muscles and the liver, and is a signaler to many other hormones in the body to increase carbohydrate burning. Insulin also has a very sparing effect on lean body tissue, meaning it helps preserve muscle, which is exactly what we are looking for. The less muscle that is used for energy, the more fat is burned up.

For people afraid of insulin, you can't get away from it. Insulin is necessary for optimal functioning of the human body. And anyhow, even the lowest carbohydrate diet will still make your body release insulin. The fact that ingestion of fat and protein still causes a rise in insulin is often ignored by low carb dogmatists.

Beef, for example, releases more insulin than White pasta – a food commonly avoided by many dieters for reasons that are not substantiated. All of this time, people have been harping on about how carbohydrates are detrimental to weight loss because they cause the body to release insulin, when in reality, insulin can be released by fatty foods with little to no carbohydrates in them. Some of the low carbohydrate foods caused an even greater total insulin response than sugary foods, which was proven in a study by Holt et al. (1997), but we will discuss insulin more in a moment.

There is another rationale behind the low carbohydrate diets. This is the idea that the body cannot store fat if insulin is not released, so by cutting out carbohydrates we inhibit our own body's natural fat storing hormone and store no more fat. Although this again sounds plausible, the reality couldn't be further from the truth. If we ignore for the moment the fact that the body *can* store fat without insulin (we have other hormones, such as Acylation Stimulating protein, which store fat in absence of insulin), we must remember that our insulin levels are never completely diminished even in a fasted state.

And even if we don't store the ingested fat, we still have to burn it off from our blood. While our body is using this fat floating around in our blood, it has no need to burn our body fat stores. So, while fat storage might be lower with a lower carb diet, our body just switches to burning blood fat instead, and the net effect on our body fat stores is the same. At the end of the day, it is still a game of energy in versus energy out.

Insulin regarding weight gain

The insulin argument fails in terms of logic, and fails in terms of practical application. I will spend a few moments breaking down the argument, and providing proof of its fallibility, so that you are left with a freedom to not only eat carbohydrates, but to eat them in any form you wish. If you want to have something loaded with sugar then feel free to do so, as it will not impact your weight loss goals when energy balance is managed. I will even provide scientific studies to back up any claims, just so you can be sure of their validity.

First we must look at how carbohydrates affect energy in; they don't - enough said. If someone eats 500 calories of carbohydrates, it is only possible to store 500 calories of energy as fat. You can't just 'magic' some energy out of nowhere. A *maximum* of 500 calories will be converted into fat, not more. And this is not including the carbohydrates which get burned there and then on the spot, or the carbohydrates which get converted into glycogen rather than fat. It is quite possible that only a very small percentage of these 500 calories are turned into fat, as most of it is converted into glycogen and stored in the liver and muscles before fat gain ensues. Even if the carbohydrate meal was very insulin spiking, this only changes the speed at which carbohydrates get converted, not the total amount.

What about energy out? Again, carbohydrates do not negatively affect energy out. In fact, they are more likely to raise our metabolism through raising many of the hormones, such as Leptin, which deal with energy regulation. So again, this person who ate a 500 calorie carbohydrate meal is safe regarding weight gain, as long as their daily energy expenditure is greater than 500 calories, which is certain.

Insulin regarding fat loss

The argument that insulin prevents fat loss is only partly true. Fat loss is occurring at all times in the body. A single fat cell cannot be influenced by insulin and lose fat, but the body as a whole can continue fat burning even when insulin is in the bloodstream. It works on a continuum; the more insulin that is in the blood, the less fat is being burned and vice versa. So if insulin levels are high in the blood it just means that *less* fat is being used for energy.

If insulin levels are lower, then more fat is being used - this is true. But the human body doesn't just completely halt fat burning in the presence of insulin. If this were true then we would never be able to use fat at all, as our blood constantly has a certain amount of insulin flowing through it. Myth demolished.

When insulin is elevated due to carbohydrates, it temporarily lowers the rate of fat burning proportional to the amount of insulin released; more insulin = less fat burning. However, although fat is no longer being used as much, neither is muscle (as insulin lowers proteolysis and gluconeogenesis - breaking down and using of muscle for energy). So what is being used as fuel for your body at this point?

Carbohydrate is being utilized and burned at an increased rate, which makes perfect sense as there is an abundance of carbohydrate in the blood at this time. The great news is that the more carbohydrates are used for energy, the less can be stored as fat. So the net effect on fat stores is exactly the same as if you were to ingest the same calories but in a low carb meal. And, as a higher carbohydrate meal will replenish glycogen stores better, it can be more advantageous to include carbohydrates in your diet, especially if you are exercising.

As explained earlier, fat gain has more to do with the total energy intake against energy outgoings. Carbohydrates, even the ones which spike insulin a lot, will not affect this balance; they could even help to improve it by increasing metabolism through Leptin boosts and other beneficial hormones. Whether energy gets stored quickly or slowly is largely irrelevant, as long as the amount of energy in or out doesn't change for the worse, which is doesn't. The only time that rate of absorption becomes relevant is for diabetics and athletes wishing to recover faster, or maintain blood glucose levels better throughout their event. As far as weight loss goals are concerned, it is not significant.

Scientific Proof

As promised, a well debated argument is nothing without a guy in a white coat nodding in agreement with a petri-dish in one hand. Here are a few studies throwing the 'fat' and 'carbohydrate' and 'refined carbohydrates AKA sugars' arguments out of the proverbial window.

Noakes et al (2006) studied the effects of an 8 week diet, everyone ingesting the same calories (1400/day) with 83 subjects participating. The subjects were placed on 3 different meal plans;

> **High carb/low fat,**
> **Mixed or**
> **Very low carb/high fat diet.**

The findings were not astonishing. Basically, the low carbohydrate group lost the same amount of fat as the high carbohydrate diet and the mixed diet. This makes perfect sense as energy balance was equal via controlling calories to 1400 per day. Interestingly both the high and low carbohydrate diets lost more lean body mass (not a good thing) than the mixed diet. Again this re-iterates the fact that being too extreme in terms of cutting out one or more macronutrients does not reap any more benefits. Worse still, it could slow down your gains and have a more detrimental result in the long term.

A brilliant study by Johnston et al (2006) placed twenty participants on two different diets for 6 weeks. Each diet consisted of the same calories (1500) but one contained a very low carbohydrate content and the other was a higher carbohydrate diet. The diets were strictly controlled. Protein remained the same in both groups (high levels) and only the carbohydrate and fat contents were varied. The results? Both groups lost the same weight and fat, with results favouring the HIGH carbohydrate group (they suffered less adverse mental and inflammatory risks). The study concluded that both diets were equally effective in reducing body weight and insulin resistance, but the low carbohydrate diet was associated with several adverse metabolic and emotional effects. They also claimed the use of low carbohydrate diets for weight loss is not warranted. Does the low carb train seem to be running out of steam yet? But this was only a 6 week study - what about longer term studies?

Dansinger et al (2005) looked at the following diet protocols for a period of 1 year;

Diet	Description
Atkins	Low Carbohydrate
Ornish	Low fat, no refined Carbs
Zone	~40% carbs, 30% fats, 30% protein
Weight Watchers	general calorie control through points system

The study showed

"No significant differences in weight loss between diets after one year"

In fact, the low carb diet lost less weight overall, completely dispelling the idea that carbohydrates cause you to get fat. Not surprisingly, the more restrictive diets of Atkins and Ornish had the lowest adherence rates, with less than 50% of participants completing the study, showing just how difficult it is to maintain a regimen that cuts certain foods out.

There are so many studies out there showing zero difference between low and higher carbohydrate diets that it could fill this entire book. But it is safe to say that, the more controlled the study is, the more the differences between dieting approaches gets 'washed-out'. Especially when you look at the composition of that weight loss.

For the sweet-tooth

As a lover of all things sweet, these are my favourite studies. Surwit et al (1997) placed 22 obese women on a high carbohydrate diet. Half were placed on a high sugar diet, the other half were placed on a low sugar diet. The diets were hypo-caloric, meaning they were putting the participants in the same negative energy balance. Most people would automatically assume that the high sugar diet would perform worse; you would be wrong. After 6 weeks, results showed no statistical differences between the diets in terms of weight loss, fat loss, metabolic rate, blood lipids and even emotional effect. Both high sugar and low sugar diets lost weight. So why would you want to cut out sweet things if you can still lose weight *with* them?

The glycemic index rates how fast or slow blood sugar levels rise in response to a food. Most people believe that foods which raise blood sugars quickly cause us to get fat. However, we know from our discussion on energy balance that it is only an energy surplus which causes us to get fat, not the speed at which that energy comes in. Is there any evidence to support this? In 2008 Aston et al. studied the effects of glycemic index on bodyweight in overweight and obese women, finding no correlation between faster acting carbohydrates (like sugar) and bodyweight when calories are the same. So even when the carbohydrates come into your blood at a faster/slower rate or insulin released is higher or lower, it doesn't mean you will get fat.

What about longer term studies regarding sugar consumption? Das et al. (2007) looked at a one year trial of diets differing in glycaemic load. 34 healthy, overweight adults were put on 30% calorie restriction (negative energy balance) for 6 months, and then a self administered plan for 6 months after. After the 12 months were complete, there were no differences found between the two groups regarding weight loss, hunger, satiety or satisfaction with the food. There were also no statistically different results regarding blood markers of health; cholesterol levels, glucose levels and insulin were equal between groups. Again, another piece of evidence destroying the sugar/carbohydrate debate.

To add to this, there are always several real world examples. Michael Phelps, American swimmer and the most successful athlete at the Olympic games in 2004 and 2008 has an insane diet. Reported to consume over 12,000 calories a day; his diet consists of chocolate chip pancakes, French toast with powdered sugar, 2 pounds of pasta, white bread, 2000 calories of energy drinks and a whole pizza, all in a day! Look at his body, this guy hasn't got an ounce of fat on him. Why? He burns more energy than he takes in; his training will manage to burn 12000 calories or more which keeps his energy balance level or slightly negative.

Mark Haub, a professor of human nutrition at Kansas state university recently placed himself on a 10 week diet. The diet was 1800 calories per day, and consisted mainly of Twinkies, powdered doughnuts, chips, sugary cereals and Oreos. Despite this, he managed to lose 27 pounds in 2 months, bad cholesterol dropped 20%, good cholesterol increased 20%, blood sugar dropped 20% and his body fat percentage dropped by 10%. Even when he went back to eating normal, his markers of health remained positive, probably as a result of the weight lost.

Chris Coleson battled his weight for years; at 278 pounds he realized something had to change. He went on a diet consisting of 1400 calories a day and in 6 months had lost 80 pounds, dropped 14 pant sizes and went from 50 to 36 inch waist. The unique thing about this diet? Every meal he ate came from a very well known burger place. Oh, he also skipped breakfast every day, something we will touch upon at a later time.

Merab Morgan, Soso Whaley, Doug Logeais, and Les Sayer have all lost significant amounts of weight eating nothing but the menu's supplied from the well known burger chain. Chazz Weaver managed to lose 8 pounds of fat, maintain muscle, increase good cholesterol and decrease bad cholesterol while following a 30 day diet eating nothing but burgers. How can these people do this? They simply controlled their energy balance while doing so.

The ironic thing is that the fast food chain in this example provides all the caloric and macronutrient values of their foods, making caloric control easier to do – this same chain often gets blamed for the obesity epidemic.

But what about the documentary 'supersize me'? All this demonstrated was the effects of poor calorie control and energy balance. Eating 5,000 calories a day for a month and not exercising will put you in the same situation, regardless of what you eat.

Would We Ever Want to Limit Insulin?

Shouldn't we try to limit our total daily insulin levels to lower our risk of diabetes? Well, yes and no. We have to look at it in context and look at all the methods available to us. There are several ways to lower our total daily insulin levels, and also several ways we can lower our risks associated with high insulin without changing the foods we eat. We have the following methods to help us

Decrease glycemic load/index of meals
Decrease body fat – again, many viable ways to do this
Increase insulin sensitivity – there are several ways to do this (exercise, fasting)
Decrease speed of absorption of foods
Attenuate the effects of 'fast' carbs through meal timing/combining with other foods (fiber, protein)

The diabetes that you are worried about (type 2) is more a product of being overweight than it is insulin production. Type 1 diabetes is genetic and we are not in control of whether we get it, and although type 2 diabetes has a genetic and environmental element to it, the main determining factor is body fat status. In fact, David Kessler (author of The End of Overeating, 2009) says that we could call diabetes an 'obesity disease' as it has such a strong correlation with level of fat stores.

For those of you clever folk out there who are reminding me that correlation does not imply causation listen up. By reversing the weights of people with diabetes type 2 through diet and exercise we can reverse or even eliminate the disease, showing that the correlation *does* imply causation. As diabetes.org.uk state in their website,

"Eating sweets and sugar does not cause diabetes, but eating a lot of sugary and fatty foods can lead to being overweight."

Implying here that being overweight is one of the major causes of diabetes type 2. The American Diabetes Association also stands by this viewpoint. If we lower our fat levels, our body will lower the amount of insulin released and *this* will improve our chances of lifelong health. While there is no guarantee of anything (as a lot is largely genetically determined), we can be assured that our chances of living a healthy, full life is greatly improved when our bodyweight is normalized or reduced to healthy levels. The great thing for you is that, through the methods presented later on in the book, we will lower our body fat levels in a way that suits you.

The next method in our list is increasing our insulin sensitivity. What this means is that we can use certain tactics to improve the effectiveness that insulin has, so as a result our body will need to release less of it to have the same effect. If insulin is twice as effective, our body will only need to release half as much. It's the same as saying

"If the exchange rate goes up and my money is twice its value, I only have to use half as much to buy the same things"

Again, the diet and exercise sections of this book will explain many tactics to improve our insulin sensitivity.

So even though we have several tactics to improve our ability to cope with insulin, don't think that insulin is some kind of enemy to be eliminated. Everything must be put into context and used wisely. For example, coffee raises insulin, but coffee has also been linked to lower levels of diabetes. So there are other things going on that we are not currently aware of. Although scientists will eventually find out the answers.

Nail in the Coffin

Recently, a few studies arose which really put the final nail in the coffin on the carbohydrate and insulin theory of obesity/diabetes.

In 2014, Soare et al. took obese, diabetic patients and placed them on a diet which consisted of 150% of their normal carbohydrate intake (over 70% of the whole diet), which is very high carbohydrate. However, they restricted energy intake to just 1900 calories for males, and 1700 per day for females. The diet consisted of wholegrains and legumes (amazingly, some people now believe these are bad for you) and vegetables. The beauty of this experiment is that it was highly controlled.

The results were astounding. After just 21 days, patients not only lost a lot of weight (6.3% of bodyweight), but their diabetes symptoms massively improved. A 6 month trial using the same high carbohydrate diet showed that, out of 16 people with type 2 diabetes, all of them managed to come off their medication by the end of the trial (Porrata et al, 2009).

How could it be possible that carbohydrates are to blame for obesity and diabetes when these people *increased* carbs in a well controlled environment and saw weight loss and improvements in their diabetes? Simple – they were in a calorie deficit.

Suggestions and Lessons

The lessons from this logic, the scientific studies and the real world examples are clear. Energy balance is, and always will be, the major key in weight management. Regarding weight loss, any diet will work as long as it puts you in a caloric deficit. But I feel that you should be free to choose how you do this, picking foods of your choice that best suit your palate and life. I am not here to sell you products or food lines. On the contrary; I think you should make your own choices.

However, you should not misunderstand the message. I am not advocating that you eat nothing but junk food, nor am I suggesting you include it in your diet. On the whole, it would be more preferential if you included foods that are classed as 'clean' or whole foods. Unprocessed foods largely contain more nutrients, such as fibre, vitamins and minerals that are important for health, as well as being more satiating. But I also understand that this is real life, and to make such a big change immediately will probably lead to diet failure. It would be better if you include the foods you wish to eat in your path to weight loss, adding in more wholesome foods as you go along.

As long as you are getting your 'calories in versus out' into a desired state and you are hitting your targets for certain macronutrients and micronutrients (all will be explained later), there is no reason why you cannot include foods that are deemed 'bad' for you. As we have seen, there is not such a clear-cut line as to what is good and bad for you; eating too much 'good food' can lead to bad health, and eating a caloric deficit of 'bad foods' can lead to several improvements in health and lower weight. It is more likely that poor energy balance and lack of certain nutrients are to blame for most of the health problems in modern society.

So, in summary, low carbohydrate/fat diets are completely unnecessary and in the long run you do not lose any more weight than any other form of dieting in calorie controlled studies. The short term extreme weight loss from low carbohydrate diets are mainly due to water losses, which are quickly regained when you momentarily come off the diet. Low fat diets again are unnecessary as it is not the macronutrient type (fat, carbohydrate or protein) you eat that causes weight gain, but it's the overall amount of energy you consume relative to your energy going out.

The main point is that energy balance is the key to controlling weight. Over-consuming fat leads to fat storage by a direct mechanism. Over-consumption of carbohydrates leads to a more indirect mechanism of fat storage by limiting fat use for energy and converting excess carbohydrates into fat. But the main thing we can take from this is that no one macronutrient is to blame for our increasing weights, it's the overconsumption of total energy.

Breakfast and Metabolism

In 2003 a study managed to link the intake of breakfast with lower bodyweights (Cho et al, 2003). There was a very clear correlation between whether a person ate breakfast and what their bodyweight was, with breakfast eaters actually weighing less. But we must remember

Correlation does not mean causation

Add to this, a study which found rats that skip a meal show a lower metabolic rate. Cue a bandwagon with everyone jumping on, unfortunately heading nowhere. It makes sense to claim that if a person skips breakfast their metabolism must decline, and this is going to lead to weight gain. Wild ideas about 'starvation response' and our body turning to survival mode circulated the media and has seeped in so strong that even most of the nutritionists and dieticians believe in stoking the metabolic fire.

Everyone with a mouth is spouting the importance of breakfast and how, if you skip it, you are doomed to be obese. "The most important meal of the day" is splattered all over the fitness magazines, healthy lifestyle gurus only fuelling this myth with more unsubstantiated 'evidence'. More studies about meal frequency and weight emerged showing a lower meal frequency causing people to eat more and then put on more weight. It was all stacking up one on top of the other, and all sounds so convincing.

But it is wrong. I will take you through the 'evidence' piece by piece and deconstruct it for you, so at the end of it hopefully this myth will be put to rest.

Breakfast = lower weight

So what about the study that linked lower body weights with breakfast eaters? Well again this is a case of making a link where there is none and then filling the gaps in later. Let us take a look at the reality of the situation.

Breakfast eaters are likely to be more health conscious people and therefore more likely to be exercisers, watch the amounts of food that they eat and generally eat better quality foods. Non-breakfast eaters, on the other hand, are not only less likely to do these things, but they are more likely to be those people who skip breakfast and then grab a bag of doughnuts on the way to work, or overindulge at lunch and dinner to make up for their lack of early morning sustenance. Also, when the study is taken, a lot of the people who are **already** overweight will be dieting and thus likely skipping breakfast, so it's not that skipping breakfast caused people to be overweight, it's the other way around.

These breakfast skippers are also likely to be the people who go on crash/fad diets and yo-yo back and forth each time wasting away their muscle and completely ruining their metabolic rate. Add to this the self-reporting of peoples' food intake is very unreliable and you have a study that doesn't really find anything useful.

Overweight people may want to look good, and in reporting how much they eat they may say that they "don't eat breakfast" in an effort to look innocent. We have all been guilty of this, distorting what we really do in order to look better in front of others. If you think you are exempt from this, you are probably one of the people that do it so well you even convince yourself of your innocence. Either way, the link that eating breakfast makes you thin simply does not stand up.

Stoking the metabolic furnace

And the idea of fuelling the metabolic fire by eating breakfast? A study looked at children and their meal patterns over a 21 year period. This study was great because it looks at how *changes* in the dietary regimens of kids affected changes in obesity levels. When you change a variable you can see if it has an effect on something else so it can give a better clue as to whether or not it is actually the cause (although, still not a guarantee).

What did this study find? After seeing a 21.4% increase in the amount of breakfast skippers, they still saw no change in overweight status. So there were still thin kids, and still overweight kids. But changing the meal patterns of kids had no change in their weights; there simply was no correlation between whether a kid eats breakfast or not and whether they become overweight. (Nicklas et al, 2004).

Keim et al. (1997) split two groups of people into large breakfast and small dinner, or small breakfast and large dinner. To make the test fair they kept calories the same and swapped the groups over half way through so everyone experienced both protocols. They found that when people ate larger breakfasts as opposed to larger evening meal, they lost less fat. This was replicated when the test subjects swapped over into the alternate role. So much for "breakfast like a king, lunch like a prince and dinner like a pauper".

Rats!

What about our rats from earlier? When they skipped a single meal their metabolism slowed; how does this apply to us? Well, rats have a much faster metabolism than humans. If a rat skips a meal, its metabolism will rightly slow down in order to preserve energy and limit the risk of it going into true starvation. It is a survival mechanism that every living thing shares and has allowed us to go through times of famine without perishing.

Humans, however, have a much slower starvation response which operates on days, not hours or minutes. If *we* skipped one meal, our body does not automatically go into starvation mode, shutting itself down, helplessly cowering at the lack of food available. Where would be the survival advantage in that for a human? As our species evolved, we would have gone through many times of feast and famine, but to be so 'quick' with its assumption that there is no longer food would actually have been detrimental to our bodies and our survival. A human that went into starvation mode and started shutting down after just one skipped meal would surely have been wiped out of the gene pool a long time ago, as it wouldn't have had the energy to go out and actually look for food in the morning.

What would make more sense is if the body created energy in the morning, in order to make that human go out looking for, hunting or gathering food. If our body created some sort of motivation (hunger), yet still supplied the energy (from fat stores) to search for food through its usual means.

This idea is actually supported by research. Many fasting studies actually show an **increase** in metabolic rate for short term fasting (up to 4 days). Like the study from Zauner et al (2000) showing an increase of 14% in resting energy expenditure after 3 whole days of fasting before it started to drop off. The results were put down to an increase in norepinephrine (a hormone which inhibits the release of insulin helping you to burn more fat). Mansell et al (1990) also found an increase of 3% in resting metabolic rate after 48 hours of fasting - again proving wrong the myth that skipping one meal (or breakfast) will slow your metabolism down.

The body also releases small amounts of Ghrelin, Adrenalin and Cortisol which help motivate us to go out and look for food. The shaky feeling you get when you are low on energy is not often down to low blood sugar levels, but small amounts of these other hormones in your blood charging you for hunting/gathering.

There is a common misconception that if you don't eat every 3-5 hours your blood sugar levels will drop dangerously and your body will start shutting down. Actually, the human body is very adept at keeping the blood sugar levels very stable. When blood sugar levels fall, our body releases the stored sugar in our liver (glycogen), and when that has gone, we can convert fats and proteins into sugar, keeping our blood levels very constant in a process called gluconeogenesis. The only time this system starts to fail is in subjects that are hypoglycaemic. In normal, healthy adults we can even complete a long run in a fasted state and our blood sugar levels are the same as when we started.

Now many people are reading this and probably worrying that they are hypoglycaemic as they feel so drained if they miss a meal. Well hold your assumptions to yourself for a moment. A recent study looked at people with supposed hypoglycaemia and found that their blood sugar levels were completely normal during these episodes. What is more likely is the psychological element of believing you have low blood sugar levels as you haven't eaten in the last few hours – it is amazing what belief can do for us, just ask any scientist about placebo's. With that said, it is important that you check with a medical practitioner if you are concerned about being hypoglycaemic.

Meal Size and Frequency Regarding Weight Gain

Arguing cases of meal frequency and skipping breakfast/meals takes us nicely into the next topic. If we are eating more frequently then generally we should be eating smaller meals and snacks. When we eat less frequently we would have to have bigger meals in order to meet our daily caloric needs. Think 3 meals of 600 calories versus 6 meals of 300 calories. Now, again, everyone is blindly repeating that big meals cause you to gain more fat/weight. Why are people saying this? Well the following explanation is what has caused the rise of this myth.

"When you eat a big meal you are putting more sugar and energy into your bloodstream, thus this causes a higher insulin response – more insulin is released. Insulin is the hormone that helps store fat and glycogen so as a result of consuming a big meal we store more fat." (anon)

Many studies have shown that larger meals or meals with higher glycaemic indexes (High glycaemic index foods release sugar into the bloodstream quicker) increase insulin levels greater. So the theory is that if we keep a lower, more constant supply of food or 'drip feeding' energy into the bloodstream we can control blood sugar levels better and keep insulin levels low causing us to store less fat. Hopefully now you are starting to see the flaws in this argument from the previous sections of this book. If not, let us go through them together.

Firstly, when you eat a big meal, it is true that *normally* more energy will go into the bloodstream and usually more quickly too (although it depends on the glycaemic index/load and combination of the foods eaten). As a result, it is true that the insulin response will be greater (but again we have seen that insulin response is not always directly correlated to glycaemic response). Also, it is true that insulin is the hormone that helps shuttle that extra energy away into fat, muscle and liver stores (it is not the only thing insulin does, actually this is a relatively small role). All sounds so convincing doesn't it? But we must push further. What about after the meal has been consumed? What about the next 4-6-10 hours? What happens to insulin then? What happens to our fat stores then?

After the big meal has been ingested there will be a large insulin spike until the food has been digested and stored, after which insulin levels will **drop** back down to baseline. What occurs next is not rocket science; it's plain obvious. The stored food is then used by the body to fuel itself for the next few hours until the next meal is ingested, starting with what is stored in the liver and moving more towards what is stored as fat.

The net effect is the same on fat stores. You may have stored fat quicker by eating the big meal, but then you've also entered fat burning mode for longer in the time between the meals. A smaller meal size with higher frequency does the same thing but on a lot of smaller levels. Instead of seeing 3 big peaks (more fat storage) of blood glucose and insulin levels followed by longer resting or more fat burning periods, we see 6 smaller spikes of less fat storage with less rest in between (lower fat burning). The end result is the same regarding insulin levels; we call it 'insulin area under the curve' and it relates to total daily insulin released.

This is supported by research from Holmstrup et al. recently in 2010. They looked at 3 different parameters, a high carbohydrate 3 meal a day pattern, a high carbohydrate 6 meal a day pattern and a high protein 6 meal a day pattern. They found no difference in the overall 12 hour insulin response for the 3 meal or 6 meal a day protocol, even though carbohydrate content and calories were equal in both. The 6 meal a day high protein condition did result in lower insulin area under the curve (total insulin) which may be useful later on in this book – but this was a result of increased protein content not increased meal frequency.

There have been studies that link decreased meal frequency with negative effects. Usually the designs of the studies have been severely flawed in many respects, comparing extremes of both variants such as 1 meal versus 20 meals a day, or many have not been calorie controlled – probably the single most important element to a well designed study. Studies have linked lower meal frequencies to increased bodyweights, but this has been a result of consuming an excess of daily calories in that lower meal frequency, not *because* of the lower meal frequency itself.

Add to this the findings by Mattson (2005) in the annual review of nutrition, showing lower meal frequencies give the same benefits to blood health markers when in a dieting state, and we have no reason to start eating every 2 or 3 hours, especially when dieting. Take another study by Cameron et al. (2009). They found that by giving people an equi-caloric energy restricted diet (basically, everyone had the same calories while dieting) it made absolutely no difference whether they spread that out in 3 meals or 6 smaller meals. In fact, when combined with other factors such as exercise, one's own preferences to meal size and other recent proposed health benefits, it can be much more beneficial to decrease meal frequency.

A meta analysis of **all** the meal frequency studies (La Bounty et al. 2011) recently reported no benefit to resting metabolic rate or to body composition by increasing meal frequency. 'Fuelling the metabolic fire' as the media would put it, does not exist. This is all you need to know.

While these myths are generally harmless (certainly not as harmful as cutting fat out of your diet), it is completely unnecessary and misleading for the general public. Eating a breakfast or eating frequent small meals is not a *bad* thing but there is no need to freak out if you miss a meal or go without breakfast one morning, worrying that your body is going to collapse into a metabolic mess. Your body is very good at keeping things going and is nowhere near as hasty to go into starvation mode as the media or supplement companies would have you believe. In fact, you will see later on that breakfast skipping/less frequent meals can actually be massively beneficial, not only to your weight loss goals, but to your overall health. But if you wish to continue eating lots of snacking meals then this is also no problem, this is The Flexible Diet after all.

Final Thoughts

So, with this section over, you should now be on your way to 'diet enlightenment'. All of those worries about meal sizes, whether to eat carbohydrates or cut them from your diet, whether to eat fat or not etc. should be no longer of any concern. You should realize that you can still eat some 'cheat foods' and still lose weight, as long as your energy balance is as desired.

The whole point of this section was to clear your mind of some of the myths and misconceptions surrounding dieting, as I personally find that most people are held back by these ideas. The restrictive nature of these myths tends to prevent people from either starting in their weight-loss journey, or ultimately sabotaging themselves as they feel they cannot stick to the strict, made-up rules, which are completely unnecessary in the first place.

Freedom is the key here, and the key throughout. The freedom to choose what you eat, when you eat it, how many meals you eat in a day, and even when you eat those meals. Freedom and flexibility will be your friend in this journey to a slimmer and healthier **you**.

Chapter Summary

Energy balance is king when it comes to weight loss. Every scientific study shows that decreasing calories causes weight loss

The types of foods you eat are largely irrelevant to weight loss. For example, carbohydrates are no more fattening than fats. Hundreds of studies have shown this

You can even lose weight eating fast food or sugary foods, as long as the energy balance is tipped in your favour. This is not to say that we *should* eat these foods, just that it can be done

The hormone 'Insulin', while currently vilified, is not a driver of weight gain directly. It cannot create an energy increase in the body without excess energy coming in

Eating breakfast does not cause you to be slimmer or fatter – it is the total daily/weekly/yearly energy balance which matters

Meal frequency does not increase metabolic rate. Whether you eat 3 or 8 meals a day is not going to make a difference to your metabolism.

Missing a meal does not put our body into metabolic decline. It would take over 48 hours of no food at all to see a lower metabolism occur

Meal size also does not affect weight gain, unless it increases total energy intake

SECTION 2
THE DIET

Chapter 3
Calorie Restriction with Optimal Nutrition (CRON)

The reasons for our rise in obesity have not been the fault of any one nutrient such as carbohydrates, protein or fat. Nor have they been a direct result of declining quality of food such as the rise in fast foods. They have simply been a result of an increase in calories ingested versus a decrease in calories expended during the day.

Now it is not to say that sugary foods, high fat foods, salty foods or any other type of great tasting food have been innocent in this whole deal. The better tasting the food the more we tend to consume of it, and if it is packed with lots of energy then it will increase our total daily energy balance and make us put on weight. But that is the whole idea, it is the excessive energy intakes (coupled with a decline in energy expenditure) that we have to address over anything else.

Diets tend to do this in an indirect way, by limiting your choice or cutting out certain foods. But we have discussed in detail the detrimental effects of these. With 'The Flexible Diet' you take direct control of the mechanism, allowing you the freedom to choose which foods *you* want to eat, as long as you don't increase your overall energy balance. With the correct plan in place it is still possible to eat foods that are 'bad' for you without going over your energy tipping point.

Swinburn et al. (2009) studied what the major drivers of the obesity epidemic were. The findings were that the average US adult consumed an average of 2400 calories daily in the 1970's, compared with 2900 calories in the 2000's. This is a massive leap in daily calories considering estimates for a pound of fat are 3500 calories. They came to the conclusion that

"Increased energy intake appears to be more than sufficient to explain weight gain in the US population. A reversal of the increase in energy intake of (500 kcal/d) for adults and of (350 kcal/d) for children would be needed for a reversal to the mean body weights of the 1970s."

If you combine this jump of calories with our ever increasingly sedentary lifestyles we can see what a mess we are getting ourselves into.

What Can We Do About This?

Our main weapon in the fight to obesity is calorie restriction. We have discussed in the last section of the book (Energy Balance) that we have to make sure less energy is coming in than is going out. But it is important just to re-iterate that message one more time, just so it really sinks in.

As long as your energy intake is less than your energy outgoings, you will lose weight. Don't feel restricted in your food choices. Try, where you can, to make more sensible food choices so that your vitamin and mineral needs are met. But as long as you are in overall calorie deficit you can make the food choices you prefer at any time. No restrictions

There is a small disclaimer in this statement about vitamin and mineral needs being met, and this is an important consideration. If you look again at the title of this chapter, it says Calorie restriction with *optimal nutrition*. This is known in the industry as CRON and has been shown to have many benefits to health, longevity and of course, weight management.

Let's delve a little more into the benefits of calorie restriction; they go far beyond pure weight loss.

Benefits of Calorie Restriction

One of the things highly associated with diabetes and obesity is insulin resistance. This is where your body is no longer sensitive to the hormone insulin, and so your body will compensate by increasing total insulin levels throughout the day.

Insulin sensitivity basically means that your body responds better to lower amounts of insulin; it is a good thing. If you are 'insulin sensitive' it means your body can absorb nutrients (carbohydrates) much more efficiently and so your body doesn't have to produce as much insulin to have the same effect. This has the knock on effect of making you more insulin sensitive and so forth.

Although many people are probably wondering why on earth you would want to be able to make it easier for your body to absorb nutrients (like fat and carbs), it is advantageous to your health. Having too much sugar floating around in your blood can lead to several negative consequences such as depression, blood pressure increases, sleepiness (or even coma), amputations, eye, kidney, heart and nerve damage to name but a few. So improving your insulin sensitivity lowers your risk of type 2 diabetes and associated illnesses.

Luckily, Calorie restriction is one of the best ways to improve insulin sensitivity, as studies by Joseph et al (2002), Goodpastor et al (1999 and 2010), Blumenthal et al (2010), Yukiko et al (2001) and Chomentowski (2009) all demonstrated.

A very recent study by (Lim et al, 2011) placed several diabetic patients on a severely reduced calorie diet. While not recommended to go this low for many reasons, the results were astounding. Markers of health improved dramatically and the majority of people in the study reversed their diabetes – after just 8 weeks on the diet. We have to remember that this study was undertaken with clinical supervision, but it offers hope to newly diagnosed diabetics and also offers us an insight into how to potentially limit our chances of getting the disease. It seems that through a lower energy intake, patients were able to lower their body fat levels and re-set their insulin producing and sensitivity.

Another indicator of insulin sensitivity is our fasting level of insulin; all the above studies showed a marked improvement in this measurement. Other markers of health include blood pressure and cholesterol levels. Although cholesterol is important and necessary for humans, high levels of cholesterol in the blood can damage arteries and are potentially linked to heart disease. High blood pressure (or Hypertension) can be an indicator of other problems in the body, but is also one of the risk factors associated with heart failure, stroke, kidney problems and aneurysms. The studies by Goodpastor et al (2010), Meyer et al (2006), Blumenthal et al (2010) and Yukiko et al (2001) showed normalized blood pressures and improved cholesterol levels when people were calorie restricted. It is probably worth mentioning that all the above studies showed improvements in weight and fat loss, obviously.

Long Term Benefits of Calorie Restriction

Although most of the above studies were relatively short term, Fontana et al (2004) conducted a study evaluating the effects of long term caloric restriction on risk factors for atherosclerosis in individuals for an average of 6 years. Comparing them against a control group, the CR group had body fat percentages averaging 9% compared to the 24% from their control group. All measures of cholesterol levels, fasting glucose, fasting insulin and blood pressure were all markedly lower in the calorie restricted than in the American diet group, even though they were similar before the study began.

In Japan, there is a tradition called "Hara Hachi Bu", which means to only eat until you are 80% full. This tradition is a form of calorie restriction in itself. Is it any wonder that the Japanese live such long lives and have some of the lowest rates of obesity? Populations with the lowest calorie diets (with optimal nutrition) have the highest rates of centenarians. In Okinawa, Japan, so many people live past 100 that there is an ongoing study of their eating habits, which also includes the Hara Hachi Bu tradition.

Why CRON Works

So how does calorie restriction work? Your body needs a certain amount of energy every day; this is called your total daily energy expenditure (TDEE). This energy is used for cells, the brain, heart, lungs, nervous system, kidneys, liver and for muscular movement and homeostasis in the body. As we have seen, we have stores of this energy in our body in forms of fat, proteins (in muscle) and carbohydrates (in the form of glycogen in the liver, fat cells and muscle cells). We maintain a level energy balance by eating the same amount of energy as we are expending through our metabolism, and if these energy requirements are not met the body must get it from some other source.

The first port of call is the glycogen stored in the liver, but after this is in decline our body switches to increased fat oxidation, which is our goal. By not supplying your body with enough energy and/or increasing energy expenditure we can break down our fat stores and achieve the weight loss we desire. When we are in a negative energy balance (losing weight) we are releasing less insulin throughout the day as a whole, as insulin responds to energy intake (not always proportionally). When our cells are not getting hit by insulin so often, they become more sensitive to it. This is the same as if you listen to your favourite song too much it doesn't have the same effect on you. But by listening to it less often we can get that old feeling back again, similar to increasing insulin sensitivity.

As stated before, our bodies are in a constant state of building up and breaking down fat stores. When we enter a calorie restricted state, our bodies are basically breaking down more fat than it is building up. Over time, this results in fat and weight loss.

How to Do It

Now comes the fun part, how to actually do this. Should you start cutting your calories to absurdly low levels in an attempt to lose as much weight as fast as possible? Why not just never eat again? The answer is that this would have the long term effect of backfiring on you in many ways, creating a plateau in your weight losses, decreasing your health, increasing muscle loss and not to mention would probably create a food crazed psychopath in yourself. There are sensible ways to do this that make it easier and healthier and give you continual improvement, rather than the extreme shortcut diets that fail more often than they succeed. Most notably a smaller more chronic calorie restricted diet.

Rather than creating a massive deficit in your daily calories, see it more as a small chunk off every day. You must see the bigger picture, you didn't just wake up overweight one day; it's a slow incremental process that creeps up on us without us knowing. The same philosophy can be applied in reverse. Be sensible about it, your body and health should be treated with respect. This is a marathon not a sprint.

Working it out for yourself

First we must work out how many calories you need in a day to sustain yourself. Then we have an upper limit of how much energy we can eat without gaining weight. Calculating your daily caloric needs is not a precise science; there are many different methods to do it. Your litmus test will be whether you are losing weight or not and whether fat mass is declining in your body. However, in order to get a basic idea of where you should start we can use the following tables.

Females

Bodytype (female)	Sedentary	Active	Very active
Petite	1600	1800	2000
Medium	1800	2000	2200
Large	2000	2200	2400
extra large	2200	2400	2600

Males

Bodytype (male)	Sedentary	Active	Very active
Small	2000	2200	2400
Medium	2200	2400	2600
Large	2400	2600	2800
extra large	2600	2800	3000
Double XL	2800	3000	3200

Please note that the above calculations are for your general daily activity meaning your work hours and what you do after work. We are not calculating exercise for this just yet. If you exercise twice, three times or every day of the week we will perhaps be adding this onto our calculations in later chapters. So this calculation could be called your Total Daily Energy Expenditure (TDEE) **minus exercise.**

It is important to understand that the above is just a guideline. Decide which category you think you come under, but don't worry if you are wrong as you can easily adjust it through the diet until you find the right amount of calories for you. Just get a basic idea of where you are now and work from that, you shouldn't be too far from the mark with your best guess.

You must also understand that everyone is slightly different and some people will have a naturally higher or lower metabolism than others. Metabolism declines with age too, so if you are a little older, then maybe choose a lower size class than suggested in the table. If you feel you are out of the realms of the table (maybe you feel you are even more overweight than the table includes) then stick to the maximum value in your gender. For example, if you feel you are a sedentary XXXXL male, stick to the sedentary double XL calories – 2800.

One other way of seeing your total daily energy expenditure is to keep a food diary for 2 weeks, noting down all of your ingested calories. Total up the weekly amount and see if you have maintained your weight, then repeat this for a second week for a more accurate reading. This does require that you maintain your weight for the week (or very close to). If you gain weight during the test, adjust the calorie estimate accordingly. This can be a little difficult, as by the time you finish reading this book you will want to start your diet immediately.

For a more accurate reading

There is a more complicated method of working out your caloric needs that would provide you with a much more accurate measurement, but it requires that you have some awareness of what your current body fat percentage is. We can work this out best using callipers (a strong recommendation to purchase a set – they are not usually very expensive, much cheaper than the more useless bioelectrical impedance devices). You can also go to your health advisor to have this worked out professionally, although I find the callipers a much cheaper and very consistent method personally.

Katch-McArdle formula (BMR based on lean body weight)
This formula from Katch & McArdle takes into account lean mass and therefore is more accurate than a formula based on total body size. Since the Katch-McArdle formula accounts for Lean body weight it is an equally functional formula for both men and women.

The formula is;

Calories needed (men and women) = 370 + (21.6 X lean mass in kg)

For example
If you are female
You weigh 160 lbs. (72.7 kilos)
Your body fat percentage is 25% (40 lbs. fat, 120 lbs. lean)
Your lean mass is 120 lbs. (54.5 kilos)
Your BMR = 370 + (21.6 X 54.5) = **1547 calories**

To determine total daily calorie requirements from BMR, you simply multiply BMR by the activity multiplier below

Activity Multiplier
Sedentary = BMR X 1.2 (desk job)
Mod. active = BMR X 1.35 (standing most of the day/walking a lot, non strenuous activity)
Very active = BMR X 1.5 (moving around most of the day/strenuous activity)
Hard labor = BMR X 1.65 (example – working on a building site)

So in our example, our woman has a job where she walks around most of the day working on a production line at a factory. The job is not particularly strenuous so she would be in the Mod. Active category. This gives her a total daily caloric need of

1547 X 1.35   =   2088 calories per day

Now if this lady exercises on top of this, the energy burned from the exercise should be added to the above total. If, through working out your daily allowance using this formula, you have come to a very different caloric recommendation than the previous table suggests, you can decide which one is better for you. Go between the two values, opt for the lowest value, or stay closer to the higher value. This diet must be right for you, as long as you are in caloric deficit you will consistently lose weight. If you are not losing weight, then drop your calories further. Just try not to be too hasty about it. Sometimes weight loss can have a slight lag time to it. Just because you didn't lose a pound this week doesn't mean it's not working. Stay patient and you will see the weight come off. We will discuss this more in depth in our periodization planning.

I've worked it out, now how many calories should I eat?

It is commonly accepted that a pound of fat contains roughly 3500 calories. I give this ballpark figure as a guideline and although it randomly fluctuates and varies from person to person in how you lose the weight, it is a good enough guideline for our simple task of weight loss. Ideally, a safe amount of weight to be lost per week is between 0.5 and 3 pounds of fat, with the higher number applying more to people who are undertaking exercise regimens and are starting with a heavier body weight.

Sure, other diets will make claims of 10 pound or more in a week. But as we have discussed, this is not fat loss but mainly water losses. Any more than 3 pounds lost per week and you are running the risk of malnutrition. Initially you may lose more weight in your first few weeks of dieting due to the aforementioned water losses, but this should level out after time and by maintaining a healthy balanced nutrient content in your diet you will limit the loss and regain of this water.

Faster is not always better

With weight loss, everyone is looking for the quicker fix – the extreme weight losses and crash diets which cause 10lb of loss or more in a week. But a few studies have confirmed that you are doing more harm than good with this approach.

Garthe et al (2007) found that athletes who had the quickest weight loss also lost the most muscle (not good) and lost the least fat. It was better to spread the weight loss over a longer period of time. Chatson et al (2006) also found that the degree of calorie restriction related to muscle loss – with bigger calorie deficits promoting more muscle loss – not a good thing.

There have been studies showing that more extreme dieting performs better, and this can be true in certain situations. In most cases, a slow and steady weight loss goal does not inspire someone as much as a "lose 10lb in 20 days" plan, and so motivation is much higher in the latter case. However, as we will see in our psychology and goal setting chapter, we can make small and steady goals seem inspiringly massive too.

In one study, participants lost more weight with the more extreme protocol. However, most of the people re-gained that weight after the trial. Extreme diets are impossible to stick to for life, so ultimately fail in the long run. We need something more flexible and something which will keep us on track for life. Like this diet.

So we should only be looking to create an energy deficit of 1000 – 7000 calories per week from our food, this will supply us with a steady weight loss. I would suggest starting at the middle part of that scale, looking to lose around 3500 calories per week.

If you are much heavier and your calorie allowance is higher, then you can afford to go more towards the 7000 calories deficit per week deficit. In the opposing fashion, if you are on the lighter end of the body weight scale it would be wiser to stick to a smaller deficit and lose weight much slower. However, in all cases I would not recommend going below a total daily intake of 1200 calories for a woman, and 1600 calories for a man per day as an average. The reasons for this are plentiful, but mainly you will struggle to include all the required vitamins, minerals and other valuable nutrients for optimal health. However, there may be scenarios presented later in the book which may drop calories below this amount for brief periods of time.

Although diets that are extreme in nature have been shown to work even in clinical studies, they are generally too painful mentally. It is much better to have a smaller deficit and lose weight slower without noticing it so much. Take baby steps and you will get where you want to in the end.

Calorie counting

One of the unfortunate things about this single most important principle is that it does require you know how many calories you eat during the day. I am not talking about working out calories to the nearest 5 or 10 calories. Even rounding up to the nearest 100 is not important. If we are making a 3500 calorie deficit per week, being out by 100 calories per day is not going to ruin your weight loss dreams, it may just make them a little less efficient/reliable.

But the problem is that most people severely underestimate their daily calorie intake. Studies have consistently shown that people who say they eat very little often 'forget' those calories from drinks, snacks and dressings etc. that can add a huge amount to your daily intake. Calorie control is a very consistently accurate way to lose bodyweight, but you must not be cheating yourself. That can of Coke you had earlier in the day, or the 3 spoons of sugar in your coffee can be enjoyed, but they also must be counted in your daily intake if you are to take control of your diet.

So the main advice here is to start a daily diary of the foods you eat. Again, consistently taking a daily diet diary has been proven over and over to dramatically improve your weight loss. The diary does nothing physically, but adherence and less self-cheating occurs when things are written in black and white. Those who were asked to keep a diary of food intake were much more likely to achieve and maintain their weight loss goals (Baker and Kirschenbaum, 1993).

This goes for any goal in life; analysis and writing down of your goals and daily monitoring are key ideas to success. There are plenty of websites that will tell you how many calories are in certain foods, and in most countries it is a requirement to state the nutritional information on everything you buy in a supermarket. Even most restaurants now provide a calorie count for their entire menu. Although these can be out by as much as 20%, do not worry yourself unless you are eating out every night of the week. The extra

100 calories or so in the meal is not going to turn you into an overnight failure (who knows, you may get lucky and have a meal that is 100 calories lower than it states). But overall the message is clear; it is becoming easier to work out your calorie intake now, especially with government initiatives to push these ideas.

Like any skill, it may be difficult at first to work out calories. But every skill that is practiced eventually becomes automatic. The first time you try any sport, musical instrument, skill etc. it is always difficult. First we have to go through it logically, then we try it and make mistakes, then we get better but we still have to think about it, then finally it becomes automatic or instinctive. These are the stages of learning for almost everything we do as an adult. If you practice calorie counting enough you can work out how many calories are in a meal without even reading packets or looking them up online, it becomes an instinct. But until you gain that instinct you must first learn by reading the labels and/or using websites to help you out.

Keep things consistent at first

One of the things that can help you is to have certain dietary staples. What this means is to have a certain consistency to the meals you eat. That doesn't mean eat the same things every single day, although you can as long as your daily staples cover a range of nutritional benefits. But try to work out some sort of meal pattern for the week or bi weekly. As long as you have certain recipes that you have worked out the nutritional information of, you can re-use these over and over so you don't have to count as much – you will have them written out in a recipe sheet or something similar.

For example, you could design 10 different 500 calorie meals that you could alternate throughout the week. Will this book suggest what to eat? No - The book is here to educate you and then let you decide what you want to eat, have fun yourself making these meals based on what you want to eat.

Calorie counting takes maybe 5 minutes out of your entire day, maximum. If you are too lazy to spend some time educating yourself on calorie amounts in certain foods you eat, do you really want to lose this weight? It eventually becomes automatic – I can tot up the calorie amounts in my head as I am walking to work. You don't have to become obsessed about every single calorie that crosses your lips; as I stated, as long as your calorie estimates are not wildly out, you will be ok. And if you are shooting for a 5000 calorie deficit in the week, being out by a few hundred (or even 1000 calories) will not halt weight loss, simply slow it down.

For those who simply can't/wont calorie count

Calorie counting is highly recommended, you are far more likely to succeed in your efforts if you do so. But I understand that sometimes real life gets in the way, or you are simply a person who is not willing to do so. If this describes you, it is a shame as such a small thing can lead to huge benefits for you. However, below describes a different way to make sure you can lose weight if you simply will not calorie count.

One of the less efficient but easier methods to use is portion control. Sometimes it can be easy enough to judge how many calories are in something by merely guessing based on the size of the meal. If you cut your average meal in half, it is simply going to have half the calories. Now, if you do this for 2 of your 3 meals a day, you can cut out 1/3 of your daily calories. This is a much simpler method to use and requires no calorie counting, however it is also much less reliable. But if you feel this could work for you then go ahead and do it. This is very easy to do if you already have certain meals that you consistently eat and know how much you normally eat. But if you do have these consistent meals it would be much more preferable if you were to spend just half an hour and work out the precise calories in each of these meals.

A method of guessing calories can be used if you are not willing to weigh things. Generally, a portion of lean meat (chicken breast, turkey etc.) the size of your clenched fist will provide 150 - 200 calories and 30-40 grams of protein. This is if it has no seasonings or dressings on it, of course. The same amount of carbohydrates (rice, couscous, oats, etc.) will provide the same, about 200 calories. The same size in fatty sources – such as butter, nuts, cheeses etc. can provide anywhere from 300-900 calories, or possibly more depending on fat content. Again, doing it this way is such an imprecise science, it would be much better to work it out, at least once with common foods you use.

Things are always much more valuable when you have quantifiable data. But it is also understandable if some people are not so analytical. Some people could also use the points systems of other diets. Usually these are a more fancy way of telling you how many calories are in the foods. The whole point is that you are eating less energy as a whole. However, awareness is key to the whole process. The more consciously aware you make yourself the higher your success rate will be.

Chapter Summary

Work out how many calories your body needs per day to maintain its weight, this is called your Total daily energy expenditure (or TDEE) but does not include exercise, yet.

Make a deficit of between 1000 and 7000 calories per week. If you are a bigger person and have more calories to work with, you can make a bigger deficit. If you are more petite and have fewer daily calories, then a smaller deficit is required. Also, the closer you are to your ideal weight, the smaller your deficit should be.

Do not go lower than 1200 calories per day for a woman, 1600 per day for a man. If your body is resisting strongly you are probably making too large a deficit.

Create a certain level of consistency with your meal plans so that you can more easily work out how many calories you are eating. For example, create 10 or so different meals each containing 500 calories so it is much easier to monitor. Be sensible, allow yourself to veer away from these staples to avoid monotony, or include new recipes every now and again to keep things fresh.

Keep a daily food log to note every calorie you eat until it becomes automatic. Alternatively (but less effectively), halve the portions of one or two of your 3 daily meals to create a 1/3 total daily cut in calories. Keep reducing portion size until you feel your body is getting lighter.

If it is not working then cut calories further per week, or be stricter on your counting. Be patient however; sometimes you are losing 'true weight' but maintaining or holding water weight. Give it a couple of weeks before you change your approach, weight loss is not always linear.

Chapter 4
Calorie Cycling / Distribution

We have looked in the last chapter at the main instrument in order to achieve our goal of negative energy balance in order to lose weight – calorie restriction. The problem comes when we are on a chronically lowered calorie intake. Every day our body is in a deficit we release hormones into our bloodstream which make us hungry and make us want to resist dieting. If you have the willpower of a 4-year-old with a juicy marshmallow in front of them, then this can lead to problems. People who have very strong willpower will be able to go through the pains associated with lowered intake of calories as they will see the bigger picture of what they are trying to achieve. Part of the battle is keeping this in mind, as we will go through later in the book with mental tools to aid in our success. This next tool however, will limit the negative impacts of a lowered calorie intake, both physiologically and mentally, helping you create a more comfortable environment with which to lose weight.

What is Calorie Cycling/Distribution?

Calorie distribution means how you portion out your calories throughout a given period of time – say every 2-3 days or every week. Calorie cycling is repeating those given periods of time over again. In the last chapter we looked at creating a weekly deficit. For example;

Woman X has a maintenance of 2000 calories per day.

Her weekly calories are therefore (7 days multiply by 2000 calories) 14000 per week.

We would like her to lose about 1 pound per week which is around a 3500 calorie deficit per week.

Therefore, Woman X's weekly calorie allowance is 10500

Our above example can choose to spread these calories out in any fashion she wishes, some days having higher calories and some days opting for much lower. As long as the weekly calorie total is less than maintenance, our above example will lose weight. Below are some examples of how our lady could choose to allot her calories.

Every day 1500 calories
1 day of 1200 and 6 days of 1550
4 days of 1200 calories and 3 days of 1900
3 days of 1200 and 4 days of 1725
5 days of 1200 and 2 days of 2250
6 days of 1400 and 1 day of 2100

The possibilities are almost endless. The first suggestion of eating 1500 every day is a very stable approach that would work. But for the majority of people it never allows them the opportunity to satisfy cravings – a vital part of any successful long term strategy. There are several diets that employ a cheat day/cheat meal strategy such as the last 2 examples (5 days of 1200 calories followed by 2 days of 2250 calories, for example, allows a person to re-feed twice a week, which could be set out as two cheat days a few days apart). You must remember that this is a controlled cheat. This means that even though we are going to indulge in our cravings we must still do it with the total weekly calories in mind. It is not a 'free for all' entitling you to gorge on as many sweet and highly calorific foods as possible with no limits. The idea still stands however, arranging your week so that you can allow for some indulgence. See it as a reward for being good on your 'low days'.

Benefits of calorie cycling

This idea works for a number of reasons, both physiological and psychological. Dieting, as we have seen, is very difficult to maintain for a long period of time. Being in a constant state of deprivation is only maintainable for a certain small percentage of the population. Even then it eventually fails and those people come crashing back to earth with a bang (and a few extra pounds).

People who lose vast amounts of weight very quickly usually end up 'burning out' and never achieving their goals. If we allow ourselves to satisfy those cravings and momentarily depart from our deprived state, it allows us to continue our diet for much longer. A person who loses half a pound a week for 10 weeks is much better off than a person who loses 5 pound a week for 2 weeks, then spends the next 8 weeks putting it all back on again. Remember the Hare and the Tortoise? The person who burned out is now the same weight, but with a deep hate for dieting as it was so painful for them the last time. Whereas the 'slow and steady' person is 50lb lighter at the end of the year.

The 'quick fix' approach will never win out in the long term. So why not take on this advice and lose weight at a smoother rate, staggering the diet so it is not constantly depriving. Depending on how you set it up, it could allow you to eat even more than your normal (maintenance) amount some days and still lose weight. The re-feeds also allow us a chance to revitalize our body with vitamins and mineral requirements not met fully throughout the week. Hopefully, if your calories never go below 1200 calories per day for a woman and 1600 a day for a man you will be able to maintain levels of all nutrients. The staggered approach makes sure that they can be topped up if there is anything lacking in your diet. However, there are even more benefits to this approach.

Alternate Day

It is recommended that you alternate the days that you have low calorie intake versus higher. Also recommended is that you never go for more than 2 days in a low calorie state as it is more likely to negatively affect your metabolism. Metabolism changes are a result of several of things; genetics, bodyweight, age, lean body mass, energy intake, macronutrient intake, vitamin and mineral levels, exercise levels, amount of sleep etc. Being in an energy deficit will also affect our metabolism, there is no doubt about that. Any form you wish to choose to distribute your calories will eventually result in a lower metabolism, whether you have a twice weekly re-feed or you maintain the same calories day in/day out. However, it seems that an alternating approach or cycling of high and low days can attenuate the decline in metabolic rate.

Fasting studies have shown that it takes up to three days of zero energy intake before we see a negative change in metabolism. Mansell et al, (1990) and Zauner et al (2000)) even showed an increase in metabolism after the same time. There are studies which show small declines also, but the evidence is mixed, and the declines are not substantial. Either way we can be assured that one or two days of low calories should not adversely affect our metabolism, especially if followed by a maintenance day or a re-feed. It is more likely that human metabolism follows a 2-3 day cycle rather than a 2-3 hour cycle as the current day media suggests. It is certainly ludicrous to propose that skipping one single meal is going to put our metabolism into lock-down.

Is there any scientific support for what I am saying? Well apart from the aforementioned studies showing potential theoretical benefits, this theory has actually been put into practice by Heilbronn et al in 2005. Subjects were put on an alternate day fasting protocol, which consists of eating nothing for one day, followed by ad libitum (whatever they wanted) the next. The subjects lost weight (2.5% bodyweight, 4% fat loss) showing that overall they were in a calorie deficit. Interestingly, resting metabolic rate did not change from baseline throughout the 21 day experiment. Also by the end of the study their bodies seemed to switch to a huge increase in fat burning and lower carbohydrate burning. Now the last sentence, although many of you probably read that thinking it is a key point, is actually not of much importance. Although it sounds flashy and beneficial, the net effect on fat stores would be the same. We may burn more fat, but we are also using less carbohydrates for fuel (and hence storing those unused carbohydrates as fat), so we will have the same results. But it could help us in terms of potentially losing stubborn fat (hips and thighs for women, belly/love handles for men) as some other scientific research has suggested of fasting.

The main point is that, through this alternate day approach to dieting, subjects were able to maintain the same metabolic rate that they had at the start of the experiment. Looking at the data and seeing that the majority of weight loss came from fat, this shows that the metabolic rate probably didn't decline due to the retention of lean body mass. It is well known that lean body mass is one of the defining elements to our metabolic rate; one of the reasons metabolism declines as we age is that our muscle levels decline through lack of use and changes in hormones. It would seem that through the massive re-feeds on high calorie days, people were able to maintain more muscle tissue. Muscles are very different cells in that they are able to take in carbohydrate energy in a one-way street. This means that once a carbohydrate has entered a muscle cell, it is there to be used only by the muscle. A chronically lowered calorie intake would eventually deplete muscle stores over time, thus losing muscle mass. It would make sense that a massive calorie re-feed would replenish muscle stores better thus maintaining muscle mass thus maintaining metabolism. Interesting.

Another proposed benefit of the alternate day approach is that, through the re-feeds, our subjects were able to consume a lot of carbohydrates. Carbohydrates seem to have a big influence on Leptin - a hormone that plays a key role in determining our energy intake and outgoings through regulation of metabolism and appetite. Leptin tends to circulate our body at levels proportional to body fat, and signals to the brain that we have had enough to eat. After a big meal, our Leptin levels raise and we become more satiated, we feel full and happy. Romon et al (1999) Showed that meals containing a high proportion of carbohydrates were able to increase circulating levels of Leptin dramatically, thus giving us some sort of explanation for why our alternate day fasting subject were able to maintain metabolic rate even though they were having days with complete absence of food.

Calorie cycling also gives many of the same benefits of calorie restriction and more. Varady et al recently (2009) looked into an alternate day approach to dieting, consuming 25% of calories on diet days followed by ad libitum (free for all) on other days. Although considered potentially limited due to the lack of restrictions on the ad libitum day (it is still very possible to overeat and more on these days), the results were very positive. Subjects lost a consistent amount of weight per week (1.33 pounds of weight loss per week) and body fat decreased significantly more than bodyweight, showing retention of lean body mass. Other health benefits occurred including lowered blood pressure, lowered bad cholesterol etc. Most importantly of all, adherence rates to the diet were very high, much higher than any normal diet leading the researchers to conclude that this method of cycling calories

"is a viable diet option to help obese individuals lose weight and decrease cardiovascular disease risk".

Is this the only study showing this? Well, as of yet the research into calorie cycling and/or alternate day fasting is not as substantial as other forms of dieting, but it is starting to get there. More and more scientists are intrigued by this form of calorie restriction as it is starting to prove to have a lot of benefits. Halberg et al (2005) studied the effects of alternate day fasting and re-feeding on healthy men and showed that insulin-mediated glucose uptake rates improved (a fancy phrase for saying lower diabetes risk) with the fasting/feasting protocol. On top of this, the study was done without a caloric deficit. If we were to add a caloric deficit to this the effects would have been even greater.

Johnson et al (2007) Studied this diet protocol on asthma patients for 8 weeks. Their findings? Participants lost 8% of their initial bodyweight, mood and energy improved, total cholesterol levels decreased, Markers of oxidative stress improved and even their asthma greatly improved. The ad libitum, or re-feed days, also seemed to halt any further losses in Leptin levels on calorie restricted days. As Leptin relates strongly to metabolic rate this is a very good sign for maintaining our metabolism while dieting.

Varady conducted another study more recently in 2011 to look at the effects of alternate day calorie cycling versus the standard daily calorie deficit. The study found that although both produced a very similar total weight loss, calorie cycling was superior in that the subjects lost less lean body mass (basically they lost more fat) prompting Varady to state that

"Intermittent calorie restriction may be more effective for the retention of lean mass".

Again, if lean mass is retained better, this will have a better overall long term effect on our metabolism as lean body mass is one of the key determinants of metabolic rate – as well as how toned you look. Many bodybuilders have also used calorie cycling in their diets to improve their fat losses while limiting their muscle and metabolism decreases; and if there is one group of people who know how to get to low body fat levels, the bodybuilders of the world are top of the pile. Bodybuilders regularly clock in at less than 5 percent body fat during a competition, having dieted down without losing muscle. Maybe your goal is not to be the next Arnold Schwarzenegger, but you can take a leaf out of their book in how to shred body fat effectively.

So we can see that calorie cycling can offer potential benefits hormonally, metabolically, physically (regarding how toned we look as a result of increased lean body retention), and psychologically through higher retention rates and cheat days to look forward to. Also, long term it could help us as we would see better results if we were to come off the diet as our metabolism has been maintained better. On top of that, advantages to asthmatics due to lower levels of inflammatory factors push the benefits further.

Psychological Benefits

We have talked so far about the physiological benefits to this approach, but perhaps the more notable benefits are psychological. Dieting is a strain on the mentality of a person as much as it is on their body. The alternate day approach enables a person to get through the process much easier. If you know that you only have one day of dieting followed by a day of eating normal, it is much easier to stick to it. When a diet is prolonged and there are no 'planned rests' from it, it is easy to lose motivation and give up completely. By staggering your calories in this manner, there is a planned rest potentially every other day, giving yourself a chance to satisfy your cravings if you wish.

This, in turn, means higher motivation on lower calorie days, being more mentally and physically prepared for them. Remembering that tomorrow is a high calorie day can also help you through a low motivation point on your down day. You can, however, choose to stagger your calories in any manner that you wish. If you feel highly motivated, why not add an extra low calorie day? This will allow you to save some calories for times when you feel less motivated. But don't do this too much or it may backfire and you lose the benefits of calorie cycling. Two or three days in a lower calorie state is the maximum recommended before switching.

You can also use calorie cycling to schedule a day where you eat more than maintenance calories one day. For example, if your maintenance calories are 2000 per day and you have one day of 1200 calories, the next day you could eat 2300 calories and it still averages out as a deficit. Cycles showing much more dramatic daily variances than this have been shown to work in our last few scientific examples.

Another benefit is social. How many times have you had a diet spoiled by a social occasion; you see no way out of it so you end up jumping in head first and ruining your diet completely. By utilizing calorie cycling, you are able to manage your own weekly calories so that you can fit these social occasions into your diet without it spoiling it. Not only does it now seem less negative, but an occasional splurge can be seen as a positive - as long as you keep your energy balance in check.

At the end of the day, a diet that lasts longer wins out over a short term rapid weight loss which is unsustainable. Losing 6 pounds in a week is not sustainable (not to mention most of this weight is water) and will lose to a more sustained loss of 1 pound per week, or even less. The problem with the traditional dieting approach is that there is never an end in sight – or that end is so far away (lose 30 pounds) that we never make it there. Take small baby steps and get rewarded for your hard work regularly and you will be sure to get there. It is the most efficient way for long term learning and for achieving our goals and dreams.

Calorie cycling is our main tool in making calorie restriction more easily achieved, and it proposes benefits equal to or above calorie restriction alone. The major reasons for diets failing are evaded or attenuated, leaving you with more flexibility. And that is the main point of this; the flexibility to choose when you diet and when you don't so that it fits into your life better.

How to Do It

So what plan of action should we take to include this idea into our regimen? It is largely a personal one, but I would certainly recommend an alternate day approach as this seems to suit mentally and biologically (which obviously intertwine). But please do not be obsessive about it. The main idea should be there to make the diet easier, not more difficult. If you would like to take 2 low days followed by a slightly bigger re-feed then go ahead. Or if you have a difficult weekend ahead of you where you know you will be eating a lot, perhaps a party or other social function where it cannot be avoided, then try to reduce your calorie intake through the week.

Below are three examples which should produce roughly the same weight loss for our example lady (who has 2000 calories daily maintenance).

Day	Example 1	Example 2	Example 3
Monday	1400	1200	1200
Tuesday	1600	1900	1200
Wednesday	1400	1200	2250
Thursday	1600	1900	1200
Friday	1400	1200	1200
Saturday	1700	1900	2250
Sunday	1400	1200	1200
Total	**10500**	**10500**	**10500**

So, in example 1, this person takes a more level approach to their diet, alternate day-ing, but never dropping calories too extreme so never feeling too deprived, and then able to have a small 200 calorie extra re-feed every other day (and 300 calories extra on Saturday). This would be suitable for someone who has an insatiable appetite when on 1200 calories a day. By increasing the low day slightly, it limits some of the cravings, but at the same time they never get to have that bigger splurge and treat themselves.

Example 2 shows a more orthodox or recommended approach. Calories are cycled every day and alternate between a clearly defined high and low day. Low days are a little tougher to get through, but with the knowledge of what tomorrow brings it is not so difficult to hold the willpower. Example 3 would be a little more difficult as there are two days of low calories in a row. However, they are separated by 2 larger re-feeds which act as a reward for their hard work and willpower during those 2 low calorie days. This can actually be a very satisfying way to lose weight, as psychologically it offers huge benefits and trains you to be disciplined with the whole process. The work/reward relationship gets ingrained and it almost becomes a game that you are playing against yourself that you will always win.

Be consistent, yet flexible

Although the alternate day high/low approach would be preferable, any way which allows *you* to function best is the way to go. Situations will occur where you will have to change your approach, don't be afraid to do so. And if you can't stick to your allotted calories then it doesn't matter. If one week you were to go higher than what you wanted it is not the end of the world.

The worst thing is to be so rigid that you cannot operate. Too many times people say something such as "Oh well, I can't stick to my diet this weekend so there is no point in me trying at all. I will just gorge all weekend and then start afresh Monday". I'm sure I have struck a chord with everyone reading that last sentence. This type of approach never wins, as something will always pop up. Just do the best you can with every week. See it as a small goal, to see how well you can stick to the week, or even smaller, see how well you can stick to the 2 or 3 day cycles you choose. If something goes wrong don't just give up. Just start afresh; you can always find a way of implementing your mistake into your weekly allotment. It is more important that you improve and get a step forward, or at the very least don't take a step backwards, most weeks. If you have this approach, you will eventually reach your target.

Notice I didn't Say 'every week', insinuating that even if some weeks stall out (as they inevitably will), you must see the bigger picture. The psychological tools promoted later in this book will help you overcome those idiotic moments where you give up, and make sure that the snowball effect doesn't happen.

Chapter Summary

Use your knowledge from rule 1 (calorie restriction) to work out how many calories you need in a week to maintain your weight (simply multiply daily calories by 7)

Work out how much of a weekly deficit you would like/could handle - take that value away from the above amount. Between 1000 and 7000 calories deficit per week is acceptable. Possibly more if you are more overweight and have a bigger calorie allowance.

Cycle between low and high calorie days. Use the high calorie days as re-feeds and rewards separated by no more than 2 days of low calories. This promotes better hormonal balance and adherence to the diet through psychological benefits.

You are free to distribute the calories as you wish, although a simple alternate day high/low pattern would theoretically be best (although everyone is different, find out what works for you). Make sure your weekly total matches a value lower than your maintenance calories for the week.

Be as consistent as you can, yet flexible. Don't give up just because you mess one day up. This weekly view of calorie intake allows you to adjust for your mistakes more easily, making it much more flexible if you are to have an 'off day'.

Enjoy your high days. Go on, treat yourself. But it is not a free ticket to an eating contest.

Chapter 5
Macros, Micros and Food Choices

The three main energy containing macronutrients are Carbohydrates, Proteins and Fats. Micronutrient is a fancy way of saying vitamins and minerals that are essential for optimal functioning of the human body. We have seen that we should include all of the above to some extent in our dieting regimen; extracting one or the other would produce more unfavourable outcomes than benefits. This section will give a brief outline of what each of the nutrients do and how they can help us, followed by recommendations for implementing into your diet. Let's take a brief look at carbohydrates.

Carbohydrates

Carbs can come in many forms - long chains of glucose molecules bound together called starches, or much simpler forms which we would call sugars (glucose, fructose, sucrose, lactose, maltose etc.). They are used by the body directly for energy, although some do not enter the bloodstream and are used by the liver to store energy for the brain.

For the most part, carbohydrates enter our bloodstream and replenish lost energy in cells throughout the body. When we have a lot of carbohydrate units in our bloodstream, our body releases hormones to help store the excess in muscles, fat stores and liver in the form of glycogen, which will be released back into the blood again in order to keep our blood sugar levels constant. Common dietary staples of carbohydrate include rice, pasta, breads, wholegrains, potatoes, oatmeal etc. We can also get carbohydrates from fruits and vegetables, although they tend to be in smaller amounts.

Carbohydrate sources tend to be very high in vitamins (in the case of fruits and vegetables) and minerals (in the case of wholegrains), or often both. They are also a great source of dietary fiber, an indigestible part of plant food that helps maintain digestive tract function amongst many other things.

Potential health benefits of fibre have been proposed, such as lower rates of heart disease, diabetes and certain types of cancers. A study of 388,000 adults ages 50 to 71 found that the highest consumers of fiber were 22% less likely to die over this period. In addition to lowering the risk of death from heart disease, consumption of fiber (especially from grains) appeared to reduce the amount of infectious and respiratory illnesses. Also, fiber consumption lowered the risk of cancer-related deaths amongst male subjects (Park et al, 2011). Does anyone want to give up their carbohydrates now? Aim for about 25 grams of fiber or more per day.

But not all carbohydrates are equal. Some are more 'empty' than others. This is a way of saying that some carbohydrate sources include more vitamins, minerals, fiber and other potential health benefits than others. For example, a bag of sugar is not going to have as many vitamins, minerals and fiber as the same amount of calories of vegetables. Does this mean you cannot enjoy a sugar in your coffee – of course not. Just make sure that, on the whole, you make better food choices in order to get more of the good stuff.

We have already discussed the speed of absorption argument in terms of sugary foods or foods high on the glycemic index, a supposed index of carbohydrate quality. Many foods that are great for you are ranked very poorly in this index, and many foods that are rated as good sources are actually very nutrient devoid. So don't worry about the glycemic index; choose the sources you are most satisfied with. Try to maintain all of your vitamins and minerals and include the other strategies in this book to improve your overall health and ability to control blood sugars.

Freedom of choice is what is going to make this diet work. We all know what we should and shouldn't be eating. Unprocessed foods, on the whole, are going to be more nutritious and better for us than processed foods. But the main goal of this diet is to improve your weight, which will have massive benefits for your health and psychology.

Carbohydrates are also important for muscle glycogen replenishment. If we are to eliminate carbohydrates from our diet then our muscles will not be able to work as efficiently, as stored levels of glycogen become depleted. This will lead to increased muscle catabolism and hence muscle loss, slowing our metabolism down in the long run. So the message is to eat your carbohydrates, have them in any form you wish as long as you are getting your vitamins, minerals and fiber.

This is not to say to eat a bag of sugar every day – if you were to do this, you would unlikely hit your fiber and micronutrient goals (as well as other things we will see). Is it possible to lose weight this way? Yes, it is; but it is not going to be healthy. While I promote the idea that sugar is not the evil that everyone makes it out to be (especially when it comes to weight management), extremes of anything can cause issues.

Fats

Fat plays an essential role in maintaining healthy skin and hair, maintaining body temperature, and promoting healthy cell function. It is also important for the digestion and absorption of vitamins A, D, E, and K. Fats are needed as they contain essential fatty acids, which as the name suggests, are essential. Fat contains a high level of energy per gram (9 calories as opposed to 4 for carbohydrates and proteins), but can and should be included in every healthy diet.

Fats have been given such a bad rap; even to this day most people associate saturated fat with poor health. Without going too much into the debate here, the data linking saturated fats to disease is spurious at best. When we look at some societies that consume high levels of fat, some of them have the best health. Almost every diet study looked at analyzing high fat diets in a dieting state produced beneficial health effects that are normally conversely associated with fat intake. As the study by Gardner et al (2007) found that even diets such as Atkins, which is a high fat and protein diet, saw favorable effects on body mass, body fat, hip to waist ratio, cholesterol levels, triglycerides, insulin, blood pressure etc. This is not an isolated case as several other studies show. Hu et al. (2011) did a meta analysis (look at lots of data) of low carb (high fat) versus high carb (low fat) diets. They found that both diets lowered weight and improved markers of health associated with cardiovascular diseases and metabolic issues.

It seems that health benefits are more a function of eating less calories total and losing weight than they are a function of what we eat. This is probably why health issues are so highly associated with obesity, and the longest living countries are the ones who maintain healthy weights (like Japan).

We have many different types of fats – saturates, unsaturated, polyunsaturated, omega 3, omega 6 etc. One thing which has been strongly linked to good health is the amount of omega 3 fats in your diet. Typically found in fish, Omega 3 oils are currently going through a boom, as more evidence is coming out showing health benefits. While too much of anything is likely bad for you, it is certain that adding some fresh fish to your diet will aid you in getting extra omega 3's. Alternatively, you could supplement with fish oils (Cod Liver Oil), although it is likely that fresh fish will provide more health benefits.

The take home message here is that fats are not bad for you. You should be including them in a healthy diet and not avoiding them. Even saturated fat from butter/milk/cheese etc. is not the devil it was made out to be in the 1980's. This is with one exception – Trans fats.

There is a big difference between saturated fats from natural sources (such as cheese, or meat) and from cakes or pastries. It goes without saying that we should include more fats from good quality whole food sources and less from processed foods.

Protein – the Magic Macro

So from the last pages we can see that both fat and carbohydrates have important benefits to our health. From earlier examples in the 'myths about dieting' section we can see that there are very few benefits from eliminating these things in our diets. So the take home message is to include everything in certain amounts. But there is one macronutrient we haven't looked at or talked about much yet - protein.

Proteins are molecules consisting of one or more amino acids. Without boring you with the technical details, proteins are needed to build and repair tissues, as well as create hormones, enzymes, muscle, cartilage, skin and blood etc.

Protein can also help us dramatically improve our weight loss, specifically from fat, for several reasons. Bodybuilders are renowned for using high amounts of protein in their diets. A bodybuilder's goals in the run up to a competition are clear - to lose as much body fat as possible while retaining lean body mass (muscle). Protein is a vital constituent in this process, as it helps support retention of muscle mass, especially while dieting.

When our body is in a dieting state it starts to break itself down, as we have discussed. The problem is that we break down both fat and muscle to fuel our energy needs. The proportions of which are determined by many factors such as genetics, hormones, use of muscles, diet, amount of lean body mass etc. While it is not important for the large majority of people reading this to maintain huge amounts of muscle, it is still very relevant.

Why do we want to retain muscle? Wouldn't it be just as efficient to lose more muscle and fat to achieve our weight loss goals? Well this is where you have to throw away the idea of weight and look more at body composition. If we improve our maintenance of muscle during our diet, this will mean that a larger proportion of our weight loss will come from fat stores specifically. What does this mean for you? Well, on top of losing more fat, you will have more muscle underneath it to support everything, meaning a more toned and lean physique.

While most of the readers of this book may not have the goal of having a Hollywood star like body (although there is no reason why not, you just need to change your beliefs), retaining as much muscle while in the fat loss process will greatly enhance your results. If your goals are to just see numbers fly off the scales, then go and chop off your leg. If, however, you wish to see your body getting more toned and tighter, then utilizing the effects of increased protein in your diet can massively help you.

    I hear you say "but I don't want to look like a muscle-head or have bigger arms" etc. Do not fret; this is not a problem for you. Notice that the last paragraph talked about maintenance of muscle, not building muscle. While we are dieting, our body will not 'build' muscle per se; we need to be in a state of surplus calories to do that. Even if we are in surplus calories for the most part, we will not become the incredible hulk overnight. Bodybuilders take many years, hours and hours of training, lots of bulking cycles (months of excess calories), not to mention copious amounts of drugs and supplements to achieve their looks. Even then, only the genetically gifted are able to build mass as they do.

    For the regular reader of this book, the best you can hope to do is ***maintain*** as much of your lean body mass as possible and tighten up the muscle that you do possess. Protein can help us in this goal. If you are a male hoping to achieve a more muscular physique you will have to incorporate bulking cycles into your plan - there are several books out there and information on the internet that can help you learn this. However, although this is not the goal of this book, it can help you in maintaining as much of that mass as possible when in the fat loss stage. In all accounts, for both men and women, this book and this idea of increasing protein can help you achieve a more athletic and toned physique while losing more weight from our fat stores, which is what everyone wants.

Give me evidence

Let's look at some studies supporting these claims.

Noakes et al (2005), found that people placed on a higher protein diet lost more fat mass than those with lower protein. This was confirmed again by Soenen in 2012 – a brilliant study which looked at lots of differing amounts of protein carbohydrates and fats for 12 months. What they found was that the higher protein diets created more weight and fat loss than any of the other protocols. Protein amount, not fat or carbohydrate amount, was the biggest predictor of fat loss.
    An analysis of all the research (Leidy et al, 2015) had this to say:

"A recent meta-analysis showed persistent benefits of a higher protein weight loss diet on body weight and fat mass"

However, we do not need these scientific studies to see this idea in action. Fitness models around the world incorporate these ideas into their diet to improve fat loss, and it is one of the key tools used when an actor or actress must get a body to 'die for' in a few months for an up and coming film.

Further benefits

What other ways does protein help us in our weight loss (or, more specifically, fat loss) goals? Protein is a strange macronutrient in the respect that it is not very efficient at being converted into fat. We have talked a lot about how weight gain and weight loss is a simple energy in versus energy out game. Protein helps us with this for a great reason; it has a much lower actual energy count than either carbohydrates or fats. Fat accounts for around 9 calories per gram, carbohydrates and proteins around 4 calories per gram. However, in order for protein to be converted into fat and stored, the body needs to first convert it to sugar in the liver and then store those sugars into our fat stores. This is a very inefficient process and during the whole ordeal a whopping 20% of the energy is lost. That means that a gram of protein is only really worth 3.2 calories. Although this doesn't seem like a lot, it can turn an intake of 2500 calories into just 2000 worth of available energy. So it is still a game of energy in versus energy out, it's just that a lot more energy is lost with protein than any other macronutrient. Energy is lost in some respect with both fats and carbohydrates too, but to a smaller extent. So a diet higher in protein is essentially lower in calories than it states. This is known in the game as the thermic effect of food (TEF).

Protein also increases our satiety, meaning we feel fuller and for longer with increased amounts of protein. A study by Wiegle et al in 2005 concluded that increasing dietary protein resulted in greater satiety levels, to the extent that subjects consumed 441 less calories per day because they simply felt fuller. Westerterp-Plantenga (2003) stated that Protein is more satiating than carbohydrate and fat in both the short term (over 24 hours) and in the long term. This study stated high-protein diets affect body weight loss positively, improving metabolism and body composition. Also, the addition of protein resulted in better weight maintenance after the diet. Moran et al (2005), Paddon-Jones et al (2008) and Johnstone et al (1996) all found improved satiety with increased protein amounts too.

Higher protein diets also tend to lower our insulin levels. As the study in 2010 by Holmstrup et al recently showed, a higher protein intake resulted in lower insulin under the curve compared to the same calories with a lower protein intake. This means that over the entirety of the experiment, total insulin released was lower overall. This means that protein could not only have more benefits for extension of satiation, but potential health benefits associated with lower insulin levels.

Protein fest

So why not eat nothing but high protein? Because by cutting out other macronutrients we miss out on all of the vitamins, minerals, fiber etc. Add on top the other health benefits of carbohydrate and fat (for example fat being needed to absorb certain vitamins) and we can see how unhealthy a diet of such nature would be. On top of that, the psychological effects of cutting carbs or fats from the diet are unsustainable, and we are more likely to gain back more water weight when coming off them. So the message and main point here is that increasing your protein intake offers several benefits to muscle retention, energy balance, satiety which, in turn, will have a greater benefit to you in terms of increasing fat loss, maintaining higher metabolism and avoiding cravings. But don't eliminate carbohydrates or fats, just increase the proportion of allotted calories to protein. Besides, an all protein diet would taste horrible.

Micros

The term 'Micros' refers to micronutrients, or vitamins and minerals. Vitamins (A-Z) and minerals (iron, magnesium, potassium, selenium, calcium etc.) are all important for our health. We all hear the news and health experts bombarding us with the idea that we should try and get as many vitamins and minerals as we can to improve our health. The government recommends 5 portions of fruit and vegetables per day, although often this is not enough. A lot of the fruits and vegetables we eat are actually not very high in micronutrients, certainly not as high as we would have instinctively believed. It is worth checking out whether you are achieving your recommended intake of these nutrients or not. There is a wealth of information out there that is accessible to all people; take advantage of this. You will probably be surprised at how few of your daily necessities you are hitting. Those 'healthy vegetables you are eating on a daily basis could be basically nothing more than water and a little bit of fiber, to which you would have to eat your bodyweight in to get anything nutritious out of it. It would be much better to choose nutrient dense foods that offer more of the good stuff with less of the calories and energy. A fresh apricot, for example, will provide you with 13% vitamin A as its main constituent, not a lot else. For the same amount of calories, Spinach will provide you with

188% of your vitamin A, along with 600% vitamin K, 47% vitamin C, 49% folate, 20% magnesium and 45% of your daily manganese needs amongst other benefits.

Some recommendations for highly nutritious foods to include in your diet are

>
> Oats,
> Flax (linseed),
> Cocoa,
> Fish oil,
> Tomatoes,
> Spinach,
> Mushrooms,
> Bell peppers,
> Broccoli,
> Carrots,
> Sweet potato,
> Kiwi fruit,
> Strawberries,
> Raspberries,
> Almonds,
> Cauliflower,
> Kale,
> Avocado,
> Potatoes (sweet and white),
> Sardines,
> Mussels,
> Liver,
> Chickpeas,
> Lentils,

These foods contain a wealth of vitamins and minerals helping you in your goal of achieving your daily needs. These foods also tend to be higher in fiber and other health protecting benefits, as well as low in calories (the majority of the list).

While a lot of fruits and vegetables may not be so nutrient dense, I am not recommending you banish them from your diet. Most fruits and vegetables are filling as they provide fiber and mass amounts of water per serving. A 500 calorie plate of chocolate is a lot smaller than a 500 calorie plate of fruits and vegetables. Almost all fruit and vegetables are low calorie and so you can eat so many of them that it fills your gut with the sheer bulk of foodstuff. This will help you in your goal of eating less energy, as it will help you stay fuller for longer. It will also assist in diluting the energy of the food you do eat, causing it to be digested slower and hence making blood sugar levels rise slower, potentially keeping you feeling fuller for longer.

So the recommendation here is to eat more fruit and vegetables in your diet. Try to include foods that are nutrient dense, like the examples on the previous page, or search for your own with the use of the internet and other sources to make sure you are getting your full quota each day. But don't immediately exclude foods that are not as nutrient dense as you thought; you can still enjoy them as part of your diet. If they are low calorie (as most are) and you like the taste of them, then by all means eat away! If you like Apricots, eat them, but understand that you may get more bang for your buck by eating something more nutrient packed. However, there could be many other potential advantages, such as anti-inflammatory properties and other benefits that we don't fully understand yet to eating even fruits and vegetables that are 'nutritiously poor', so don't throw out the apricots yet.

How to Do It

How do we implement the above strategies into our diet? How much of our daily intake should we allow in the form of carbohydrates, fats and proteins? Although these are all very good questions, at the end of the day it is down to you. How much of your muscle mass do you want to retain, what foods do you like the most, what foods help keep you satiated longer, how much exercise do you do, how far away from your ideal bodyweight are you, is it important to you that you keep your body tone? This is The Flexible Diet, and for it to suggest you ***must*** do this or that would be to detract from its goal of becoming 'your diet', one that suits you.

For example, if you are vegan it is pointless to suggest you maximize your protein intake, as the type of protein needed to support muscle mass comes mainly from animal products. Although many vegetarian dishes can potentially have high protein amounts, the type of protein is not of the same amino acid profile as animal protein. Although higher protein potentially could have better satiating effects (such as tofu protein) it is unlikely to have much of an effect on your muscle retention.

The overall goal for the majority wanting to include this idea in their diet is to increase the amount of protein in their diet. Any increase above normal will show beneficial results for the majority. Below is a rule indicating how much protein you will need to eat per day to maximize results, although allow yourself to be flexible.

Your ideal bodyweight in pounds X 0.8 – 1.2 grams

So for example, our example lady is 160 pounds but would like to be 130 pounds. She can decide to eat between 104 grams or 156 grams of protein per day. In deciding whether to opt for higher or lower amounts of protein there are a number of things to take into consideration;

The more sedentary you are in daily life, the lower amount of protein you need

If you are not worried about retaining lean body mass (you should be), a lower protein intake is ok.

The closer you are to your goal weight, the higher your protein requirement

The more exercise you do, the higher your protein requirement

The higher intensity your exercise is, the higher your protein requirement

The more lean body mass you wish to retain, the higher your protein requirement

If higher protein intake leaves you feeling fuller for longer, as it does with most people, then increase your protein intake to the higher levels.

Although you can go below the recommended 0.8 grams per pound of ideal bodyweight, it would be much more beneficial if you stayed within this range. I would not recommend going higher than the 1.2 grams per pound of ideal bodyweight, as most research has shown it is no more beneficial (unless in certain extreme examples). It will also cut into our daily allowance of carbohydrates and fats which are also both necessary. For the majority of readers, 0.8 gram per pound of goal bodyweight would be more than enough, and you will find it is actually quite a lot of food.

We can get our protein from sources such as lean beef, chicken breast, turkey, ham, tuna, low fat milk, cheeses etc. Different sources have different amino acid profiles so it is best to mix it up every once in a while. Some proteins digest faster, some slower, some have a combination of fast and slow digesting proteins, such as milk. But if you vary your sources occasionally you will get all of your necessary nutrients and avoid monotony in the diet. You can choose lower or higher fat options – it's up to you. But make sure you stick to your daily/weekly calorie goals as closely as possible.

For example

Our lady decides to eat 125 grams of protein per day

This is equivalent to 500 calories (125 x 4 calories per gram)

She is allowed 1200 calories on low days, 2000 calories on high days

This entitles our example lady to decide where she 'spends' her extra 700 calories on low days, and extra 1500 calories on high days. She could split it evenly between fats and carbohydrates, or have a more carbohydrate or fat heavy diet. Her carbohydrate sources could come from anywhere she likes, but foods such as oatmeal, cereals, whole-grains, fruits and vegetables provide more vitamins, minerals and fiber.

Regarding fat sources, although trying to limit trans-fats is a good idea, don't over-obsess about it. Try to include more 'good fats' in your diet such as Flax seed (sometimes called linseed) which is also a very good source of fiber, and/or fish oil supplements or eating fresh fish. Uncooked olive oil drizzled over your food can also increase your amount of good fats, although watch the calorie count. Try not to cook food in fats. Instead, use non stick pans and low calorie sprays or fruit juices to get the food cooked, and then use fats in your dressings, such as a balsamic vinaigrette. By not cooking with fat you preserve the healthy benefits of them and lower overall calories – allowing you to make the most of your dressings and sauces.

Examples

To help you understand some food choices, I have placed some example foods here with some calorie guides and protein amounts.

High protein foods

Food	Calories Per 100g/3.5oz	Protein
Tuna (canned)	110	25
Chicken breast	110	22
Turkey breast	110	22
Low fat beef (ground)	130	20
High fat beef (ground)	330	15
Liver (beef)	130	20
Lean Pork Loin	110	20
Salmon	140	20
Sardines (canned, tomato sauce)	180	20
Eggs (whole)	143	13
Eggs (whites only)	50	11
Beef jerky	400	33
Milk (whole)	150/cup	8
Milk (skim)	80/cup	8
Whey Protein powder	120/scoop	25
Lentils	350	25
Chickpeas (Garbanzo beans)	360	20
Kidney beans	330	25
Tofu	145	15

All of the above are raw values (uncooked).

We can see that most sources are roughly the same, with lean sources of meat being around 110 – 150 calories per 100 grams, and offering around 20-25 grams of protein for that amount. Eggs are surprisingly low in protein – you would need a lot of them to reach your daily protein requirements. For vegetarians/vegans, we have a few sources available to us in Beans, lentils, tofu and chickpeas

Low calorie, high nutrition

It is a good idea to know a few very low calorie, highly nutritious sources of foods. This allows us to eat a lot more food while keeping the energy balance in our favour. By filling up on these foods, you will be able to save some calories for the occasional treat – and it will also help you when you're on your low-calorie days, as you can add more diet bulk with these foods.

Food	Calories Per 100g/3.5oz
Apple	50
Strawberries	30
Red Bell Peppers	30
Blackberries	40
Spinach	20
Mushrooms (white)	20
Kale	50
Cauliflower	25
Sweet potato	80
White potato	70
Tomatoes	20
Broccoli	35
Carrots	35
Asparagus	20
Lettuce	15
Cucumber	12

Don't be frightened to eat these in large amounts. Forget about standard portions – be greedy. You will often find me eating half a kilo (over a pound) of strawberries in one sitting. It satisfies my sweet tooth, and is packed with vitamins and only 150 calories. I will also often load my plate up sky high with mushrooms, spinach, peppers and cauliflower for around 200 calories – and then pour a nice sauce over the top for taste. This way, you can fill up on crazy amounts of foods without going the wrong side of the energy balance.

High Fiber sources

Food	Calories Per 100g/3.5oz	Fiber
Raspberries	50	6
Blackberries	40	5
Kidney beans	330	25
Lentils	350	30
Chickpeas (garbanzo beans)	360	17
Wheat bran (1 ounce/28gram)	60	12
Oats	360	10
Avocado	160	7
Cocoa (unsweetened) 1 oz / 28grams	80	8
Cauliflower	25	3
Flaxseed 1 oz / 28 grams	150	8
Bran cereal	270	30
Broccoli	35	3
Carrots	35	3
Parsnips	75	5

Fiber will help to fill you up, and has also been associated with many health benefit and help controlling blood sugars.

Chapter Summary

Increase your amount of protein to between 0.8 and 1.2 grams per pound of your ideal bodyweight. For example, if you wish to be 140 pounds, aim for between 112 and 168 grams of protein per day. Try to make sure your protein comes from mixed sources, but animal products are best for lean body mass retention.

Once your protein requirements are met, the rest of the calories are yours to split between fats and carbohydrates **as you choose**. Try to severely limit trans - fats, although don't be obsessively strict about it. Feel free to treat yourself with whatever you like as long as it fits in with your macronutrients and total calorie intake.

The quality of the diet as a whole, not each individual food, is what counts. If your diet is 70-90% highly nutritious, it is ok to have that chocolate bar. Fill your diet with the recommended foods and more.

Increase your amount of fruits and vegetables in order to get your vitamins and minerals required for optimal health. They provide a lot of bulk from volume of water and fiber increasing satiety by slowing down the digestion of foods, all for a low amount of calories.

Try to include more fiber in your diet from increased fruit and vegetable intake, and also from whole-grains or flax seed.

Get a non stick pan, use low calorie sprays, fruit juices or vinegars to stir fry your vegetables in order to cut down on total daily calories.

Make sure more of your fats come from good sources such as flax seed, oily fish, olive oil, nuts etc.

Do not exclude what you wish to eat, include everything as part of a healthy diet. Try to include more of the 'good stuff', but always enjoy your food.

Chapter 6
Exercise

The dreaded words uttered by many, practiced by few. Before you run for the hills skipping this chapter, read the following statement.

15 minutes per day of exercise is more than enough

Ok, now that we have got that out of the way we can digress.

Undoubtedly you already know that there are many benefits to exercise with regards to your goals, but to make it clear they are summarized below. The reason I choose to highlight and summarize the benefits before we talk about them is simply to keep you interested and maybe even motivate you to exercise. I want to sell it to you.

The benefits are;

Increased Fat loss

More toned body (better shape)

Better health

Better maintenance of weight through improved metabolic functions

Who wouldn't want any of the above? Normally people associate exercise with hours upon hours of running on the treadmill, a very boring procedure for most. What if I told you that you can achieve all of your weight loss and health goals with just 15 minutes per day (or equivalent)? While it may be necessary for Olympic athletes to train for hours each day, we can achieve great results with much less exercise. We are looking for an exercise regimen that is efficient, effective and can be done with the minimum of fuss without cutting into our daily lives. I understand that most people don't have hours to devote to exercise, but luckily this philosophy is unnecessary. Not everyone can find 2 hours to run on a treadmill amongst their daily chores of looking after the kids, cleaning the house, shopping and cooking etc. However, there is no excuse for not finding **15 minutes** a day on average. In fact, more beneficial would be to do 30 minutes every 2 days, which will be explained further.

Sustainability

An effective training regimen is not only one that works, but one that can be sustained for life. A regimen that includes 2 hours of weight lifting a day followed by an hour of cardio may provide success (it will probably also provide overtraining), but it is simply not a regimen you can keep going for long. The majority of people will get burned out mentally and physically in a very short space of time.

While your motivation is high you will feel it is no problem, but just like every other 'New Years resolution maker', you will find yourself quitting in no time. This is the exact same philosophy as our diet – if we take an extreme viewpoint, it may provide short term success, but it is set up to fail because of its lack of long term outlook. A diet which provides one pound of weight loss per week for a year is infinitely better than a diet that gives 10 pounds of loss in the first week, yet is too restrictive to stick to for longer than 2 or 3 weeks.

Our exercise regimen must be set up so we can see constant small improvements every day - the hare and the tortoise. For a movie star who wants to get into shape for a role, or for an athlete competing, they may have insane amounts of training. We have all seen the stars transform their bodies very quickly, but it is often not continued after the role has been fulfilled. We want to keep our training going continuously, so we need to do something that is not so much of an unpleasant task, or something that is quickly over and done with so we can get on with our day.

Benefits of exercise

How does exercise benefit us? In scientific studies, adding exercise to our diet and weight-loss plan consistently shows improved results. In studies by Goodpastor et al (2010), Blumenthal et al (2010), Chomentowski (2009) and Dube et al (2008), adding exercise caused a **greater loss of fat** and **less lean body mass** losses. This is old news however, and I could cite a hundred studies showing the same. What this means for you is a more toned physique, as well as lower numbers on the scale. More lean body mass preservation means you have more muscle supporting your body, so your body looks harder, more shaped, more defined and wobbles less. Having more lean body mass also (as we have described in the last section) will maintain your metabolism better, as greater lean body mass acts as an extra food store, so less of it goes into fat stores.

How does exercise do this for us? One of the main mechanisms is by nutrient partitioning - meaning that ingested energy is directed towards replenishing the muscles rather than fat stores. To understand this, we first have to visualize what happens when we exercise. As our muscles are being worked, stored energy (in the form of glycogen) is used up creating a 'hole'. This is called 'exercise induced glycogen depletion'. After we have exercised, more of the food we eat is directed towards filling this 'hole' in our muscle energy stores.

The beautiful thing about muscle energy stores is that it is a one-way process. Once carbohydrates have entered a muscle cell it is there for good until it is used directly by the muscle. The reason for this is that muscles lack the enzyme responsible to pass sugar back into the bloodstream, so the more energy that gets directed to the muscles, the less there is to be stored as fat. Also, when we are between meals, the stored energy in muscles cannot be used to fuel our bodies; as a result, our body taps into fat stores more. So not only do we maintain/improve muscle function, keep our lean body mass full and toned, but we end up storing less fat and burning more as a result.

Muscles can also absorb blood sugars independently of insulin, meaning the body doesn't need to release as much insulin - great news for lowering our total daily levels of this hormone and decreasing our risk of diabetes. With lower fat levels, increased muscle levels and lower levels of insulin, we can see that exercise boosts health in many ways. Lowering blood pressure, cholesterol levels, fasting insulin, glucose tolerance, and insulin sensitivity have all been found by Goodpastor et al (2010), Blumenthal et al (2010), Chomentowski (2009) and Dube et al (2008).

Ryan (2000) looked at the effects of combined diet and exercise on older adults and found the following;

"Several studies report that bodyweight loss increases insulin sensitivity and improves glucose tolerance. In addition, the insulin resistance observed in aged persons can be modified by physical training. Longitudinal studies indicate significant improvements in glucose metabolism with aerobic exercise training in middle-aged and older men and women. Moreover, the improvements in insulin sensitivity with resistive training are similar in magnitude to those achieved with aerobic exercise. The improvements in glucose metabolism after bodyweight loss and exercise training may in some cases be partially attributed to changes in body composition, including reductions in total and central body fat. Yet, additional changes in skeletal muscle, blood flow and other mechanisms likely interact to modify insulin resistance with exercise training. Lifestyle modifications including bodyweight loss and physical activity provide health benefits and functional gains and should be promoted to increase insulin sensitivity and prevent glucose intolerance and type 2 diabetes mellitus in older adults"

So in basic terms, by losing weight (specifically body fat) and exercising, subjects greatly lowered their chances of developing diabetes. This came via improved insulin sensitivity via all the metabolic changes associated with combined exercising and dieting. Solomon et al (2008) found that by combining exercise and dieting they were able to increase fat use, and as a result decrease the fat mass and maintain muscle mass of the subjects. This resulted in a reversal of insulin resistance (the starting point for diabetes) and improved Leptin sensitivity. O'Leary et al (2006) also found exercise alone decreased fat mass, while maintaining muscle mass. They also managed to reverse insulin resistance, which was associated with the changes in body composition, in particular Visceral fat.

Types of Training

Resistance training, or training with weights, sends a message to our muscles to stay put. Normally when we diet, our body will burn a certain amount of muscle as well as fat. Through exercising, the electrical impulses sent to our muscles gives our body a signal to limit breaking down for energy. If our muscles are being used, they are still deemed by our body as valuable to us, so our body holds on to them. However, if our muscles are not being used, our body will catabolize (break down) this muscle and use it for energy, meaning less fat is lost. Just look at a person's arm after they have their cast taken off. As their arm has been immobilized for a few weeks, you can see that their muscles have shrunk in that arm. As stated, the more muscle that is used for energy, the less fat is used – not a good scenario. But it can be minimized or prevented with the use of resistance training. So with all the benefits of exercise alone, we should now be extremely motivated to start.

There are two main types of exercise we will discuss in this chapter - Resistance training and Cardio (cardiovascular training). The main goal of our training is the maximum retention of lean body mass, with a side goal of creating a caloric burn. But we want to achieve this with the minimum of fuss and the minimum of time investment. So what type of training is the best to achieve these goals?

Resistance training

Resistance training is overcoming some sort of force by applying an opposing force; basically this means moving weight around. There are so many different ways to resistance train – we can use our bodyweight, we can use dumbbells and barbells, elastic tubing, kettlebells or just plain dragging things around. Resistance training is one of the more efficient methods to burn the most energy in the shortest period of time, therefore it is very helpful towards our weight loss goals.

In 30 minutes of resistance training, you can burn more than 200 extra calories. Energy burned from exercise means a greater energy deficit in our body, ultimately meaning more weight loss. So to make our exercise program as efficient as possible, we should include some sort of resistance training. It is more effective at challenging our muscles than most other forms of exercise such as cardio; the more stimulation (through higher intensity) that a muscle receives, the more chance you have of maintaining that muscle. And the more muscle you maintain through a calorie deficit, the more fat you will ultimately lose.

Many people avoid weight training as they fear they will bulk up and look muscly. While this is a worrying concern for most women (ladies prefer to stay feminine), you have no need for concern. In order to actually build muscle, you need to be consuming an excess of calories - which isn't a problem for us as we are on a diet. You also have to understand that building muscle is a very difficult process; you don't wake up one day looking like the next Mr Olympia. The best that you can hope for is high maintenance of the lean body mass you currently possess. For ladies, you don't have the hormones that men do, or the genetics necessary to build huge amounts of muscle.

A lady undertaking a resistance training program ends up looking very svelte, toned and even more feminine. The Hollywood stars do not get their toned physiques from hours of pounding on the treadmill; the 'secrets' they use are hidden in the iron of a dumbbell. In the initial stages of training, you may experience some 'newbie gains', which is an affectionate term used to describe a toning of the existing muscle. But do not fear that you will build huge bulging biceps; this is not going to happen during the diet. A study Teixeira et al (2003) found that resistance training provided more beneficial effects to fat mass and retaining of muscle mass than hormone therapy in postmenopausal women – but no one ended up building muscle, simply retaining existing levels instead.

For men wishing to achieve a more muscular physique it is a good idea to start on a muscle building diet (much higher calorie) once your weight loss goals have been achieved. It is possible to lose fat and gain muscle at the same time (over the period of a week or month for example), but these diets are very complex and should be undertaken once you get closer to your desired goal, if you wish. But the message for ladies fearing the bench press is not to worry; you will only get a more feminine physique by employing the tactics laid out here.

Why resistance training over cardio? Resistance training is not only better at retaining lean body mass, but your metabolic rate is elevated for many hours afterwards; we call this the 'afterburn'. A recent study by Fatouros et al (2009) found that although total energy burned was lower in high intensity exercise, resting energy expenditure (metabolism) remained elevated for much longer afterwards (72 hours compared with 42 hours). And we are not talking about a few calories here or there - they burned hundreds of calories more compared to baseline. On top of this, most of this extra energy was burned from fat, as Wu et al (2006) also discovered! So with resistance training, we are burning more calories even at rest, with more of those coming from fat stores.

Heden et al more recently (2011) confirmed findings that resting energy expenditure is elevated for up to 72 hours post workout with resistance training. More interestingly, they found no difference between 15 minutes of exercise versus 35 minutes, highlighting that you don't need to spend hours in the gym to boost your metabolism. So, although it would be more preferential to do 30 minutes or so of exercise (you will burn more energy from the extra workload in the gym), if you only have 10-15 minutes on your hands, go ahead and do a short workout. It is massively more beneficial for your metabolism than not doing it at all. Kirk et al (2009) even found a minimal resistance training regimen of 11 minutes was enough to chronically elevate resting energy expenditure, so now you have no excuses!

Everyone has 11 minutes 3 times a week.

Cardio

Cardio (short terminology for cardiovascular system training) is an exercise at a lower intensity, usually 60% or so of your maximum heart rate, which is generally sustained over a longer period of time. Running on a treadmill or spending time on a cross trainer are examples of cardio that we generally think of. These exercises challenge the cardiovascular system in a way that forces it to improve so that we can increase our efficiency of oxygen use. Our heart gets stronger and more efficient, lung function improves as a result of physical adaptations and we are able to make more use of every breath we take, allowing us to perform activities longer without becoming as tired. It also has an effect (albeit much smaller than resistance training) on maintaining lean body mass and improving strength.

Cardio, unfortunately, has in the past been hailed as the holy grail of fat loss. The reason for this absurd notion is that, during the exercise itself, you burn a greater number of calories from fat specifically. But, like much of this information, we have to see it in the context of the bigger picture; the bigger picture is the net effect over the course of the day. Although weight training creates less of a dent on fat stores during the actual process of lifting weights, the burn of total energy is much greater. When we eat our post exercise meal, more of that energy is directed (partitioned) towards the muscle, leaving less energy to be stored as fat. So although less fat is burned *during* the actual exercise, a lot less fat is stored in the hours afterwards, and so the net effect on fat stores is improved. Using cardio burns fat directly, but then more of the food we eat after the exercise is stored back in our fat stores. The net effect is a higher level of fat than if we had done the same workout using weights.

So if cardio is so poor at burning fat, why should we even bother to include it in our regimen? The short answer is that you don't have to if you don't want to, although by including it you can have some added benefits. Adding cardio is another method of burning more calories, meaning that if you include it, you can reach your weight loss goals quicker. So even though cardio is not the most efficient way to burn the most fat and improve your body composition, treat it as a supplement to aid you. Cardio also offers us benefits above and beyond simple fat loss. On top of the improved function of our heart and lungs, Cardio helps improve blood pressure, glucose tolerance, insulin levels, CAD risk, bedroom performance and thus mood.

How to Do It

Resistance Training

How you structure your workout for optimum efficiency will vary depending on your starting level; If you are a more experienced sportsperson, then you can continue with your current activities or add some of these moves if you wish. Many people reading this book may already be a bit more experienced in the gym, and that is great. If you already have a more advanced routine, feel free to continue with that. As always,

Consult your physician/medical practitioner before completing any of the advice suggested here. Make sure you get a full

physical to ensure you are fit enough to complete the following workout.

It is also important to state that you should perform a full body warm up before attempting any of these exercises. A warm up would include some light jogging on the spot, some general body movements such as arm circles, torso twists, knee kicks etc. Some very light and short stretching, and going through the exercise with some lighter weights at first can also get the blood pumping to the muscles, lowering your chance of injury and preparing your body both mentally and physically for the work ahead. If you feel you are highly unfit, it is probably better to start with cardio exercises until your fitness level improves to the point you feel ready for resistance training. Another option would be to gradually progress into this regimen, slowly increasing intensity over time. You should always be pushing yourself to some extent in order to improve, but not to the extent that you cause injury or harm.

Firstly, we need to look at the exercises we should complete. The exercises presented here are called compound movements and they include many muscles at the same time and more of the bigger muscle groups. The bigger the muscles used (and the more of them), the more energy is expended; perfect for burning lots of fat and retaining lots of lean body mass. We will not be conducting any useless crunches, hip abductors, arm curls, or girlie Swiss exercise balls. Save those exercises for the time wasters (you can include them as part of this regimen if you have more time but they are unnecessary for our goals).

It is highly advised to consult a personal trainer at your local gym so they can direct you on the techniques to minimize the risk of injury. Just one session with them going through the exercise list would be enough and wouldn't break the bank, although if you would like to get a more personalized plan for yourself then it can be a great way to start. Beware however, a lot of personal trainers and fitness experts will tend to either produce overly complex routines to justify their 'expertise', or give you something so weak that it barely works you. This exercise routine is simple, yet very effective.

Bench press

This exercise is a staple in every good fitness regimen. It uses primarily the pectoral muscles (chest), front deltoids (shoulders) and triceps (back of the arm, or bingo wings as they are affectionately known). To a lesser extent, they also involve the abdominal muscles (stomach or abs) and back muscles for stability. All of which are very big muscles, all of which are expending a lot of calories.

For the bench press, we will basically lie with our back on a bench, or alternatively on a bed with a number of pillows underneath our back so our upper body is elevated from the bed. Start with a dumbbell/barbell in each hand close to our chest (as shown in photo). From this position, simply press the weight towards the sky while keeping your back against the bench. Do not lock out the arms, keep a slight bend in the elbow to maintain tension on the muscle. Now lower the weight slowly to the start position and repeat.

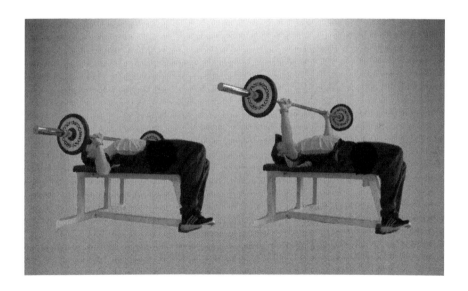

Lunge

This exercise involves the leg and glute (butt) muscles, lower back, shoulders, biceps, and upper back muscles to some extent.

To do this exercise, start in a standing position with a weight in each hand. Step forwards and bend your front leg to 90 degrees (see picture). Push backwards with your forward leg until you are back in the starting position. Repeat.

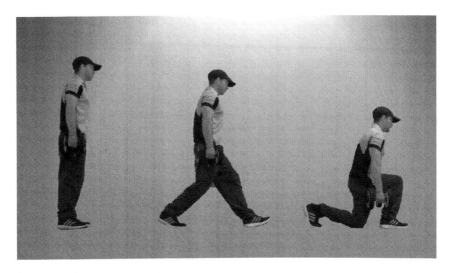

The options you have for this exercise are to stay with the same leg, exercising it until you are completed and then working the other leg in the same fashion afterwards. Or you can alternate the leg for every repetition. If your shoulders give up first – as in you can no longer complete the dumbbell raise portion of the exercise, continue with the stepping forward until you have reached your goal repetitions.

Squat

The squat should be a staple in every exercise regimen; it works our butt muscles, lower back and leg muscles. We can start with bodyweight squats and move to weighted squats as we get stronger and our technique improves.

Start in a standing position. Next, bend your knees and lower your hips down and back as you tilt your spine forwards from the hips. Try to keep your knees over your feet during the entire movement, and keep your lower back straight (which will feel like you are sticking your bum out).

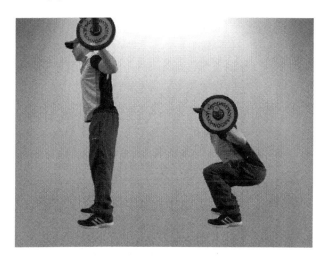

You can also do an alternative version with dumbbells. This would see you squat down into the start position with your hands and the weights by your sides. We then push up into a standing position, before repeating the movement.

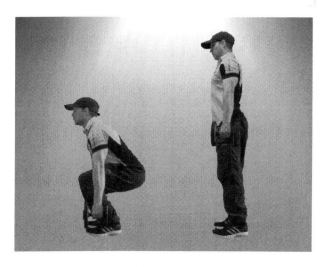

Deadlift

A deadlift works almost every part of the body, from legs, butt and lower back to our upper back and shoulders. Also, as it is one of the exercises we can become strongest at, we can burn a whole load of calories in a short period of time.

Start with a barbell on the floor in front of you. Squat down and grab hold of it. Keep the barbell close to your shins. As you lift up, keep your lower back straight and butt out – feeling as if your chest is high. After getting into the upright standing position, drop the barbell and start again.

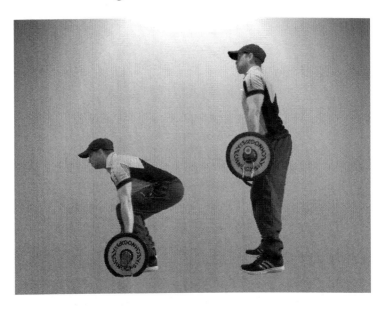

Bent over rows

This exercise works our arms and upper back muscles. If we do it in a standing position, we also work our legs and lower back.

Grab hold of a barbell or EZ bar (the one which is Zig Zag shaped. Bend your upper body forwards, keeping your lower back straight. Pull the barbell towards your chest, then lower it back down again and repeat.

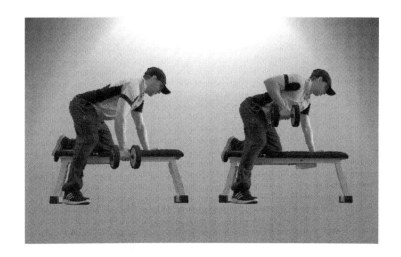

Pull ups

We have all done these – they work our upper back and our core muscles too, as well as our arms. Simply grab hold of a pull up bar (you can buy them for your house which fit in the door frame), and pull yourself towards it. Try not to swing your body, use a controlled movement.

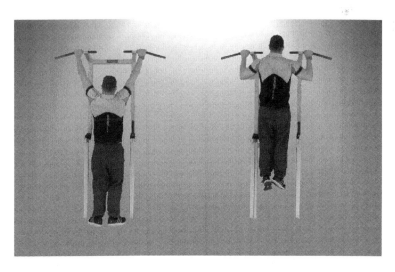

Burpees

Stand up straight, then get down into a squatted position with your hands on the floor. Kick your legs back to get into a press up starting position. With your hands still on the floor, kick your legs back into the squatted position before jumping up back into your starting position.

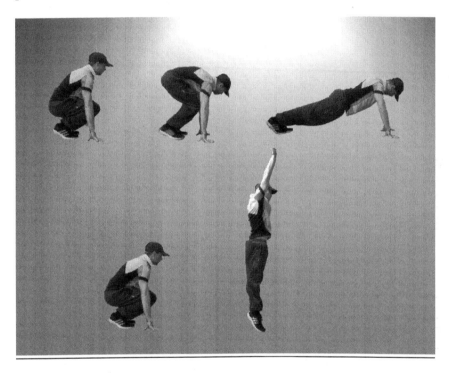

The Program

For purposes of completing the exercise regimen, the above exercises are split into 2 groups. This helps by offering a little more variation from workout to workout, and allows a bit more recovery for certain muscles. Some of you may notice that it is split into a predominantly upper body/lower body split.

Group 1	Group 2
Bent over row	Lunge
Pull ups	Squat
Bench press	Deadlift
	Burpees

Progression

In order to have an effective exercise regimen, we must gradually progress it as we improve. This will ensure that our muscles are challenged enough to be maintained, and that the total amount of energy we burn stays high.

The term 'Repetition' means the number of times you repeat a movement. A 'Set' is a certain amount of these repetitions. For example, a set of 10 repetitions means you complete the 'move' 10 times. If you are to do 10 repetitions, then rest, then complete 10 more, this is termed as 2 sets of 10 repetitions. Below is an outline for how you should continue.

Month	Repetitions per set
1	20-25
2	15-20
3	10-15
4	8-12

You may notice we are doing progressively *fewer repetitions* per set as we move forwards. While this may seem counter-intuitive, what you don't realize is that we will also be adding **more weight** and resistance over time. So, even though you will be doing fewer reps, the exercise will be more challenging and intense.

In the first month, we will use a weight that we can comfortably perform 20-25 repetitions. If we can perform more than this, we should increase the weight/resistance (take it easy on your very first week). If you tire fully before you reach 20 repetitions, then lower the weight until you can stay within the range. After the first month, your body should be well adapted to this training load.

We will increase the intensity in month 2 by increasing the weight a little; you know that you have increased the weight enough if you can no longer reach 20 repetitions. If you fail before a count of 15 then you have increased the resistance too much. The same applies for month 3 and 4 - keep increasing the weight or decreasing the weight until you stay within the desired rep range.

Pushing yourself

By month 3 and 4, if you are not reaching your desired repetition range, before you lower the weight you should first ask yourself if you are pushing yourself hard enough. This shouldn't be easy by this point. Your heart should be pumping, you should be sweating and your muscles should be burning. Do not hurt or injure yourself, but make sure you are challenging yourself enough. Remember, the more you challenge yourself, the higher the amount of energy burned and the more fat you will lose.

During your exercise session, one set should take around about a minute to complete. After you have done one exercise, such as bench press, allow yourself around 2 minutes to recover before moving onto the next set, so this totals about 3 minutes per set including the working part and the rest. As a beginner you should start with just 2 sets of each exercise. So for each exercise group (4 exercises total), it totals 24 minutes of your time. If you have not enough time one day, then either complete the exercise day on a different day or do just one set (round) of each exercise. This would be just 12 minutes out of your day, not including warm up.

After 4 months of training (well done if you are still with us), cycle months 3 and 4. By keeping our training consistent for a month at a time we allow our body to adapt positively to the workload. By cycling the rep range, we challenge our muscles in a different way and thus keep our improvements continuing for longer. In order to keep the muscles challenged in a different way, and to avoid a little bit of monotony, you should also change the exercise that you start with within the group. For example, if one month you start your group 1 training with bench press, followed by squat, followed by pull ups, then next time you are in that cycle, change the order to pull ups, followed by bench press, followed by squat.

Rest

It is important to receive enough rest so that the muscles can fully replenish and recuperate. Make sure you do not complete the same exercises on consecutive days. The exercises are split so that they allow the muscles to recover, or they are worked in a different way. So ideally complete exercise group 1 followed by group 2, and allow 2 or more days before repeating group 1 again. So your week would look something like this

Day	**Training**
Monday	None
Tuesday	Group 1
Wednesday	None
Thursday	Group 2
Friday	None
Saturday	Group 1
Sunday	None

In between weight training sessions, you can choose to include cardio if you have the motivation, or if it fits your goals. As far as cardio is concerned, try to do it in more enjoyable forms, such as playing a sport like tennis, golf, badminton, squash, hockey, soccer, football etc. Any other activity you wish can equally suffice – rock climbing, rowing, cycling, athletics, swimming etc. As long as the activities are not boring to you, as the major determinant of you succeeding in your goal achievement is to keep motivation high. Nothing dwindles motivation quicker than a routine you hate or dread to undertake.

Cardio

If you are to start running, as a rank beginner you should start with walking 10 minutes a day, gradually increasing it to 20 minutes a day. If you are comfortable with this, increase the intensity of those 20 minutes by speeding up – switch to speed walking/Nordic walking, and then jogging. If you are at the stage where jogging is no longer challenging you enough, you can alternate between bursts of high paced running (sprinting for 20 seconds) and jogging. Try to increase the total distance run in the 30 minutes rather than increasing running time. This is a form of cardio called HIIT – or high intensity interval training. This has been shown to be a very effective way to burn a lot of calories in a shorter period of time, as well as being more likely to increase metabolic rate post-workout.

By taking this progression you ensure that your leg muscles, ligaments, tendons and cardiovascular system are ready for the impact of the training. By limiting to 20 minutes maximum, you are much less likely to mentally burn out, although if you are a more experienced runner and enjoy it then you can do a routine more suited to you. However, understand that it is not a vitally important part of your success, merely an added supplement.

Calories

As you perform exercise and burn calories, we can then add these calories into our weekly calorie total. Be warned, however, exercising doesn't burn as many calories as you may think. It would be tempting to pile on the exercise in an attempt to burn more, but this is the wrong way to go about it. See exercise as creating a small weekly increase in calorie expenditure, but having greater benefits to your partitioning of weight loss (fat versus muscle).

Below are some values of calories burned during typical exercises. Adjust the values as you see fit – calories burned can be highly dependent on your training status, how vigorous you exercise, the amount of weight lifted etc. Also, if you weigh more, an exercise may burn a different amount of calories. Generally, the more you weigh, the more calories you will burn when doing things such as walking – so (in this case) pick the higher values in the range.

Exercise	Calories burned /30 mins
Light exercises – resistance training, walking, golf etc.	100-200
Moderate exercises – resistance training, swimming, tennis, rowing, running, elliptical trainer, aerobics etc.	200-300
Intense exercises – Advanced resistance training, HIIT, jump rope etc.	250-350

We see that resistance training falls into all 3 camps – depending on how vigorous you exercise. As you go through the first few months of training, stay within the first range (but towards the upper end of it). When you start dropping the reps and increasing the weight in later stages, you may start to enter the 'moderate exercises' group.

Intense exercises, such as jump rope and HIIT, burn far more calories than other exercises. However, as they are so intense, you may only be able to perform these exercises for a maximum of 15-30 minutes. They might make a nice addition if you wish to change things around or add more variance to your routines, but don't start killing yourself doing hours and hours of intense exercises (if that is even possible) in an attempt to burn more calories. Which is easier - cutting out the 300 calorie chocolate bar, or doing half an hour of jump rope?

On the other hand, activities such as golf may have a lower caloric burn, but they can be sustained for much longer (typically 4-5 hours per round). This means that a round of golf can burn quite a substantial amount of calories (over 1000).

Exercising should be there for the health benefits, fuel partitioning benefits and muscle preservation, with the calories burned being a nice supplemental benefit. If you do 3-4 sessions of moderate resistance training per week, this could account for around

800-1000 calories burned per week. When working out your weekly caloric burn, you should now add this exercise induced deficit to your total. For example,

If your daily caloric needs to maintain your weight are 2000 calories per day.

This totals 14,000 calories per week

If you burn 1000 calories per week via exercise, this brings your total weekly caloric expenditure up to 15,000 calories.

Simple. Again, our chapter on calorie restriction tells us how much of a caloric deficit you should make in order to create a sustainable amount of weight loss, and our chapter on caloric cycling show us how you can spread these calories through the week.

Burnout

While it would be possible to create a decent sized caloric burn during the week by doing mass amounts of exercise, this may not be the best option. For example,

Person A does 30 minutes of resistance training, 3 times per week, burning around **600** calories.

Person B does 90 minutes of resistance training, 5 times per week, burning around **3000** calories.

While person B creates a much bigger deficit in calories, you have to ask yourself if it is really worth it to you? If slogging away in a gym for close to 2 hours a day in order to create an extra 2400 calorie burn (around half a pound of fat) seems like a good trade-off, then go ahead. However, for most people, we want to do the minimum amount which is required of us to improve our lean body mass retention during dieting. This will mean that most people should fall under the category of Person B. Essentially, if the thought of going and doing your exercise sessions fills you with dread, you are likely going to burn out and give up in the long term. Cutting them to short but effective sessions (30 minutes of resistance training) means that it will not cut into our lives.

It would be much better if you did the minimum resistance training amount for your goals, yet found other activities which you enjoy and don't feel like you are exercising – such as golf or tennis or badminton. You will be able to stick with these activities for much longer. Doing 3x30 minute resistance training sessions a week and playing 3 rounds of golf could make a nice 3600 calorie weekly deficit. As always, it is your choice if you do more than the minimum requirements and become person B. However, if this is at the cost of you sticking to the diet and exercise plan completely, then it is simply not worth it. Decide what you can manage realistically with your lifestyle, and go with that. But try to stay above the minimum amount (3x30 minute resistance training).

Chapter Summary

Resistance train 3-4 times a week for 10 - 30 minutes (or as much as you can do, but no more than 1 hour). Do not exercise so much that your motivation diminishes; short and intense sessions are more effective in the long run.

Use exercises which employ the bigger muscles and whole body as they are more efficient at burning the most amount of calories. Start with lower intensity at first, especially if you are a beginner. Gradually increase the resistance and intensity as you progress.

Start with 2 sets of 20-25 repetitions. As your body adapts and gets stronger, increase the amount of weight lifted. By your 4th month, you should be lifting a weight that is so heavy you can only get a maximum of 12 repetitions before tiring completely.

Rotate the exercises perhaps once a month, so that you start your exercise session with a different exercise.

If you are going to do cardiovascular exercises try to do it in the form of sports/activities such as golf, tennis, swimming etc. to make it less tedious. Complete cardio on your low calorie days. If you enjoy running, by all means include it in your regimen.

Preferably keep your cardio sessions to no more than 30 minutes also. Instead of increasing time completed, purely increase the intensity and speed that you run to cover more distance in the same time, possibly by alternating between high speed running and jogging.

Work out roughly how many calories you burn through exercise in the week, and add that to your weekly calorie total.

Chapter 7
When Should I Eat?

There has been a lot of mis-information/mis-representation regarding this topic in both the scientific literature and the media. Diet books claiming that there is an optimal time to eat foods (or certain foods) have been around forever, and the media hasn't helped - claiming miracles in meal frequency and supposedly increasing metabolic rates through meal frequency/timing manipulations. The human metabolism has been likened to a fire which we have to keep stoking (via frequent feeding) to keep it burning brightly. But is there any truth to this? What if these ideas are based on weak scientific evidence, and there is just enough contrary evidence which hasn't been made as popular?

The aim of this chapter is to take a look at the evidence, and then use this information to enable us to create flexibility in our diet which can serve us. At the end of this chapter, you will feel liberated and free to eat when you desire.

Meal Frequency

How many times have you heard in magazines or on Television that you "must eat 6 times a day to keep your metabolism revving"? This idea has been so pervasive that it is now mainstream thinking. It must be much easier for companies to sell you 'snack bars' and supplements if you have to be constantly stocked up with titbits of food – heaven forbid you accidentally miss a meal and go into a metabolic coma.

However, the evidence for this fact is very weak. Most of the studies looking at meal frequency have produced neutral results (meaning that it doesn't matter how often you eat or when you eat).

The few that have shown a positive effect for meal frequency (higher being better) have been flawed in some way – using very strange protocols and/or not matching food amounts.

This myth of a higher meal frequency being better has been especially pervasive in the fitness industry, where gaining lean body mass and maximizing fat loss has been the goal. As a result of the idea that "more is better", fitness enthusiasts everywhere are carrying around several Tupperware containers filled with many bird-sized meals, obsessing over when their next feeding is. I have personally experienced this myself, and I know how detrimental that type of thinking can be, and how freeing it is understanding the truth. So, what is the truth?

3 meals or 6?

I think most of us grew up on the idea of 3 standard meals – Breakfast, Lunch and Dinner. Yet it has become more popular recently to add smaller more frequent feedings and snacks. So does eating more frequently really increase our metabolic rate? Does eating the same amount of food over smaller meals help us with blood sugar?

In 2010, Holmstrup et al studied the effects of 3 meals versus 6. This was a highly controlled study, and lots of samples of blood were taken throughout to maintain accuracy. They found that the total insulin levels for the 3 meals a day pattern were the same as for the 6 meals a day pattern – debunking the idea that bigger, less frequent meals necessarily causes a big sugar/insulin dump. In fact, total blood sugar was higher in the more frequent meal plan – they had smaller blood sugar spikes, but their blood sugars remained more elevated throughout the day. They also found that increasing the percentage of calories as protein improved both blood sugar and insulin responses, which fits in nicely with our chapter on Macros.

But that study only looked at some blood and hormone responses – what about metabolism? Bellisle Et al (1997) reviewed the scientific literature and found the following;

> *"A detailed review of the possible mechanistic explanations for a metabolic advantage of nibbling meal patterns failed to reveal significant benefits in respect of energy expenditure. "*

Also,

> *"More importantly, studies using whole-body calorimetry and doubly-labelled water to assess total 24 h energy expenditure find no difference between nibbling and gorging."*

So, as long as the total amount of energy eaten is the same, the metabolic rate will not significantly alter by splitting that food energy up into more frequent but smaller feedings or one big meal. This was further confirmed by Verboeket Et al (1993). They fed people either a 2 meal a day pattern or a 7 meal a day pattern (with same food energy amount), finding no difference in energy expenditure or average daily basal metabolic rate.

Cameron et al (2010) also found that when diet calorie amounts were the same, there were no differences between 3 meals versus 6 meals in terms of weight loss, lean body mass or fat mass. The evidence is stacking up; Nibbling or gorging – your choice.

What about Protein?

Lots of people, especially those in the fitness field, often ask me the question;

> *"But, what about protein? I heard that you have to take small, frequent amounts of protein to build muscle"*

While the majority of people reading this book will not be concerned too much with maximizing muscle gains, it is still an important consideration for those looking to stay as toned as possible by retaining as much lean body mass throughout the dieting process.

This myth has come about by people looking at short term research. Typically, protein supplement companies may have purported the benefits of smaller more frequent protein feedings (for obvious financial reasons), citing research looking at protein synthesis rate over 4-hour time scales. One of the biggest studies responsible for this misunderstanding was when Moore et al (2009) found that 20 grams of protein created no bigger a response to protein uptake rate than 40 grams of protein. This then led into the idea that more frequent feedings of 30 grams or less is more beneficial.

However, the study was severely flawed. It only lasted 4 hours and looked only at protein uptake (synthesis) rate. The issue with this is that (just like a bank account) the amount of protein retained is a product of uptake and losses. In protein terms, we would be looking at synthesis (increase in protein) versus catabolic rate (decrease in protein). In 2012, Deutz and Wolfe looked at the research containing synthesis and catabolic rates and concluded

"There is no practical upper limit to the anabolic response to protein or amino acid intake in the context of a meal"

Luckily, most of the studies which have had adequate daily protein amounts have shown no benefit to a more frequent meal pattern. And this fits in nicely with our chapter on Macros – one of the main tenets of The Flexible Diet is a higher protein intake. With our adequate amounts of dietary protein, we will have more flexibility as to when we eat that protein.

Arnal et al (2000) fed subjects protein in either a pulse pattern (one big protein amount and a few smaller amounts), or a more spread pattern (equal amounts throughout the day). They found no difference with protein retention between the groups. This study was also conducted with elderly people, and the group with the less spread protein pattern actually retained more whole body protein. So, are frequent protein feedings really that important?

Stote et al (2007) looked at an intermittent fasting meal pattern, where subjects ate one big meal a day with all their protein versus 3 meals more spread out (same energy). As expected, the bodyweights of the groups remained the similar, but the one meal/day group actually saw modest improvements in fat mass and muscle mass.

Eating Late at night

As a person who never really liked breakfast but loves to eat big meals late at night, understanding this really made me happy.

The myth here is that, as your metabolic rate starts to slow at night (due to decreased energy expenditure from less physical activity), any food you eat will be more likely to be stored as fat, as you are not burning it off. While it may be enticing to believe this idea (it sounds plausible), let's look at the logic.

If we look at weight gain as a product of energy in versus out (at every study shows is true), it shouldn't really matter when we put that energy in. If I have a bank account which has outgoings of 10,000 dollars in a year and income of 10,000 a year, the bank account will balance regardless of when the expenses and income happen. Whether I get paid monthly, weekly or even yearly will not make a difference to the end account number, as long as outgoings remain the same.

Is this backed by any research? Well, in 2011, Sofer Et al. studied the effects of a diet which had the same amount of energy, the same ratio of protein/fats and carbs, but the carbohydrate amounts were either

Evenly distributed throughout the day
Provided as a bulk amount at dinner

As predicted by logic, both groups lost weight as they were in a caloric deficit. However, the group which ate most of their food late at night actually lost more weight and more body-fat. Now, some would argue that eating late at night should surely now become the 'thing to do'. However, it is important to see that both groups lost weight, and that going with the protocol which suits you and fits with your lifestyle would be best for long term results.

I suppose this myth came about when Keim et al (1997) produced a study looking at bigger meals in the morning versus the evening. This was a tightly controlled study, and it showed that the late night eaters lost less weight.

"Wait", I hear you say. Doesn't this contradict the previous study? Well, yes and no – look deeper. The late night eaters actually lost **more fat** and **less muscle** – a great combination. However, as muscle weighs more than fat (per energy density), the morning eaters lost more weight – even though it was mainly muscle loss and not fat loss.

Meal Skipping

This title is almost too taboo to even speak. For years, the idea of missing or skipping a meal has been met with gasps of shock and horror. Surely this is completely unhealthy and against everything you have ever read in a fitness magazine, how could I possibly make reference to it?

It has been common wisdom that meal skipping will result in your metabolic rate dropping/crashing. This will reduce the amount of energy which gets burned, halting your chance of successful weight loss. But is there any scientific backing behind the idea that your metabolism comes to a screeching halt when we miss a meal?

Put simply, no - in fact, several studies have shown the reverse. In 2000, Zauner et al showed that even 3 full days of complete fasting actually increased metabolic rate by 14%. In 1990, Mansell et al also found that 2 full days of fasting marginally increased metabolic rate. So, if skipping food entirely for 2-3 days doesn't affect your metabolism negatively, skipping a single meal is not going to have any effect.

But, why would we skip a meal? Well, by taking away one of your meals, you are able to cut a significant amount of calories out of your day. If you typically have a 700-1000 calorie lunch, removing that from your diet can create a huge dent in your daily intake. This means that you can essentially eat as you normally would for the rest of the day, so you don't feel as if you are constantly dieting. Think of it as a "one-third day diet".

This can serve a significant mental advantage over traditional dieting methods, where every single meal is reduced in size. It can be much easier for a person to eat normally for breakfast, skip lunch and then have a normal dinner, rather than taking the usual view of dieting constantly throughout the day.

Obviously, this method is not for everyone – it is simply presented here as an option. Some people may not have the willpower to be able to do this, or may not be comfortable with going without food. However, the human body can last without food for a surprisingly long time and still function perfectly well, as we see in cases of people fasting for days and still going about their daily life. So skipping a single meal may be a viable option. Indeed, during Ramadan, people skip food for the entirety of daylight and get on with their lives just fine.

Which meal to skip?

The next question on your mind is "If I am going to cut out a meal, which one should it be"? This is a question ultimately only you can answer, and it will deal largely with how you personally react to food. For example, some people would find it incredibly difficult to go without breakfast, as they may 'need it' to get their day up and running. Other people may not be able to go to sleep without a hearty meal in their stomach. I also see the complete reverse, with many people able to comfortably skip breakfast and not feel any issue at all, with other people able to sleep well without having a big dinner. You will already have an idea of which camp you fall into – or you could also experiment with skipping lunch instead.

It is important to realize that your body will actually train itself to respond to what you decide. If you start to skip breakfast, for example, at first it may be a little uncomfortable (although, sit tight – you are going to eat as normal again for lunch and dinner). However, after about a week, your body starts to realize that it is not getting breakfast and starts to function better without it. You even lose a lot of your desire to eat at that time.

This effect happens because your hormones start to regulate in a different way to accommodate your normal meal pattern. A hormone called Ghrelin typically makes us hungry, and also typically gets released around 1 hour to half hour before we normally have a meal. So, for example, if you normally eat at 1pm every day, your body will start releasing Ghrelin at around 12pm. If, however, you don't eat breakfast on a more consistent basis, your body will train itself to that meal pattern and you won't release Ghrelin at those times. Your body will also set up other hormonal changes to enable you to function better during those times without food – such as an increased ability to use internal energy sources for energy (aka fat).

But, isn't skipping breakfast bad for you?

We have already covered this in our earlier chapter on dieting myths. However, to re-iterate here, no it's not. We have covered that metabolism does not crash when we skip one meal, and any studies reporting benefits to breakfast have usually been purely correlational.

Anecdotally, there is a large following of fitness enthusiasts who consistently skip breakfast – they call it intermittent fasting. Many of these people are reporting great responses to cutting out breakfast, including better health, wellbeing and physical shape.

If we go back to our study by Keim et al (1997), remember that this highly controlled study showed late night eaters losing more fat and retaining more muscle. Martin et al (2000) also looked at eating a high energy breakfast versus a low energy breakfast. In the low energy Breakfast, they consumed just 100 calories – basically nothing. Yet, (after no weight changes were seen between the groups) the author concluded;

"Results of the Study do not support the current advice to consume more energy at breakfast"

Meal Replacement

The idea of meal skipping can be a scary and dramatic one for most people. I suppose we have been so conditioned to eat at certain times that the thought of going outside of that regimen scares us. But we see animals in the wild surviving with less regular meal patterns (especially hunting animals, which may have to go for days without food at a time). So it would be ludicrous to suggest that we humans are unable to miss a single meal – it simply doesn't make sense on an evolutionary level. However, I do understand that it is a quantum leap for most people, so here I will suggest a less dramatic form.

Meal replacement refers to swapping one of your daily meals with a smaller, less caloric dense meal. This is simply a spin-off from meal skipping; but rather than eliminate a meal completely, we are simply going to reduce its caloric content. For example, you may have a normal Breakfast, a reduced size Lunch, followed by a normal Dinner. Again, by reducing your Lunch from 800 calories to 300 calories, we can cut out that 500 calories which could lead to a nice sustainable weight loss.

This also allows us to still fill up at lunch time. With the right food choices, 300 calories can actually be a decent sized Lunch. By replacing your normal sandwich with an apple, a banana and a protein shake, you can increase your protein consumption for the day (as discussed earlier), as well as reducing daily calories.

Again, we can have flexibility in which meal we reduce in size. If you typically could go without Breakfast, why not reduce it simply to a protein shake? Perhaps you would prefer a quicker and smaller lunch when you are busy through the day and not thinking about food? What about going to bed on a lighter Dinner? Use personal preference as your guide. However, if you are going to replace one of your daily meals with a smaller version, make sure that the food you eat offers a bigger bulk per calorie – such as fruit, vegetables, leafy greens etc. in order to fill your stomach as much as possible.

Calorie shifting

An advantage of meal skipping or meal replacing is that we can start to shift daily calories around as we see fit, which offers us the ultimate in flexibility. For example, if you prefer to eat a bigger dinner, why not shift some of the calories around during the day to accommodate this, eating a smaller breakfast and lunch to accommodate the increased dinner size?

This is actually my own personal preference; I don't eat breakfast, and haven't done for about 7 years. I then have a light lunch, before doing my exercises after work and having a much bigger post-workout dinner. This suits my personal preference and my lifestyle, and there could also be some other potential benefits to this way of eating (as we will find out later).

I have also had times where I have eliminated breakfast, had a much bigger lunch which satiates me throughout the day until I have a lighter dinner before bed. Again, being The Flexible Diet, the choice is yours. The main thing you must realize is that you have plenty of freedom when it comes to your meal patterning, meal size, meal frequency etc.

How it fits in with Caloric cycling

In our chapter on Caloric Cycling, we discussed the idea of alternate day dieting, where you cycle higher calorie days with lower calorie diet days. This essentially turns the diet into one which is much more sustainable, as your feel as if you are only dieting half of the time. By combining calorie cycling with the above ideas, we can have many effective ways to create a caloric deficit without the usual constant deprivation of a typical diet.

For example, you may be alternating days of higher and lower calories. It is then possible to eat as normal on your higher calorie days, and simply use meal skipping or a meal replacement on your low calorie days. See the below tables for three examples of possible meal patterns for a person with an average daily caloric goal of 1650-1700/day (when dieting).

Example 1 – The Light Luncher

Meal	High Calorie day	Low calorie day
Breakfast	300	300
Dinner	800	300
Lunch	800	800
Total	1900	1400

Example 2 – The Breakfast Skipper

Meal	High Calorie day	Low calorie day
Breakfast	0	0
Dinner	1000	600
Lunch	1000	700
Total	2000	1300

Example 3 – The Feaster

Meal	High Calorie day	Low calorie day
Breakfast	300	400
Dinner	300	0
Lunch	1200	1200
Total	1800	1600

The possibilities with this are almost endless. While I would tend to stay relatively consistent with your decided pattern, don't be frightened to mix it up and try something new every now and again to keep the diet fresh. You may stumble across something which works really well with you.

Nutrient Timing

Nutrient timing is a way of describing *when* we eat certain foods in relation to exercise. For example, does eating protein before training have an effect on how much fat we gain/lose, and does having carbohydrate after training increase muscle retention and aid in minimal fat gain?

Scientists have tried to answer these questions for many years and have come up with some principles to help us with our weight loss goals. While the majority of information is directed towards sportspeople looking for optimal performance, the rules can apply directly to our own goals of improving fat loss and increasing muscle retention. The information here will be put simply. Sometimes there can be a tendency to overcomplicate these things, but in reality it is not such a minefield of opportunities. The human body has a wonderful way of adapting and working with what we give it, and so although most of the strategies in this section are not vital, they may offer a big psychological bonus on top of the physiological benefits which are supportive to your success.

Energy Pre-Workout

On our days where we are working out, it certainly may be beneficial to have certain nutrients timed around these workouts. For example, many people may wish to not workout on a completely empty stomach, which is understandable.

However, with that said, there are plenty of fitness enthusiasts currently doing the intermittent fasting protocol (usually where they skip breakfast) and working out while completely fasted. Many are reporting workouts of similar or even higher quality, although much of this is likely a placebo effect.

In essence, it is up to you what you decide to do. Possibly, timing your meals so that you have something in your bloodstream as you workout may be more comfortable for you, although it is not a pre-requisite, and you will likely achieve similar results with your body composition whichever method you choose.

Post-workout protein

This area has been the cause of much debate over many years. Many books and philosophies have been built solely on the premise of an optimal post-workout feeding routine. While some of it may have credence, much of it is simply extrapolating incorrectly from study data.

Most post-workout nutrition has looked at shorter time scales immediately after the workout – whereas we should really be looking mainly at the longer term effects. For example, many studies claim that eating protein immediately after your workout is vital for success. Many of these studies were severely flawed and didn't match protein amounts, or used negligible amounts of protein in both cases.

In 2013, Aragon and Schoenfeld did a review of the meal timing literature and found that;

"even minimal-to-moderate pre-exercise EAA or high-quality protein taken immediately before resistance training is capable of sustaining amino acid delivery into the post-exercise period"

So, if you have taken a meal containing protein before your workout, you don't need to run and grab a protein shake immediately after the last bead of sweat falls, as the nutrients from your pre-workout meal will still be sufficiently supplying you.

However, that is not to say that protein timing is completely irrelevant. Crib and Hayes (2006) found a greater increase in lean body mass after 10 weeks where subjects had pre and post workout protein, compared to the same nutrition that was separated away from the training by 5 hours either side. This shows that delaying workout nutrition too long either side of a workout bout may result in less than optimal results.

This may become important for those of us partaking in meal skipping. If you were to "meal skip", it might not be best practice to do so in a way which leaves your body without nutrients around your workout. For example, if you were to have a normal breakfast, skip lunch and work out, then not eat again until late in the evening, this may be less than optimal. Also, if you were to skip breakfast and exercise in the morning, if your next meal is not until lunch, this may also produce suboptimal results. Indeed, Aragon and Shoenfeld did state

> *"in the case of resistance training after an overnight fast, it would make sense to provide immediate nutritional intervention--ideally in the form of a combination of protein and carbohydrate"*

So, the overall message here is that protein consumption before or after a workout should optimize lean body mass retention. However, as long as you eat something before you workout, you don't have to obsess over eating a meal immediately post-workout. And if you are doing fasted exercise, post-workout protein ingestion may be more important (do it within 1-3 hours of working out), although understand that this is simply optimizing lean body mass retention and should not be obsessed over.

Carbohydrate timing

When we exercise, we create a hole in our muscles (a glycogen deficit) which gets filled back up when we eat enough carbohydrates. This process is called glycogen re-synthesis. Eventually, given enough carbohydrates, our muscle glycogen stores will re-fill, so it is not so important to be worried about the timing of carbohydrate intake.

However, for athletes, this may be a more important concern. For example, if you have to undertake several exercise sessions using the same muscles within 24 hours, the timing of carbohydrate intake is quite important. It would be better to intake the majority of your carbohydrates around and in between the two exercise sessions so that the majority of the carbohydrate goes towards fuelling the exercise and replenishing muscle stores.

However, the majority of people reading this book are not going to be elite level athletes, and your exercise days will typically be separated by several days where replenishment can occur. So, *when* you eat your carbohydrate may be less important.

With that said, muscle insulin sensitivity is greatly improved following exercise bouts. This can allow our muscles to preferentially store any carbohydrate we eat, as opposed to going towards liver glycogen replenishment. So, practically, if you are dieting and undergoing a lower carbohydrate version of The Flexible Diet, it may be beneficial to eat the majority of your carbohydrates after your workout, when it is more likely to be stored in muscle. Chronically, this may help with muscle retention and workout performance. There may also be other reasons for doing this.

Stephens et al (2007) showed that taking a large carbohydrate meal immediately after exercise greatly improved insulin action (think of it as insulin effectiveness). This was shown even when all the energy was replaced that was lost during exercise. Three protocols were undertaken where the carbs were given before, immediately after, or 3 hours delay post-exercise. The 'Pre' protocol increased insulin action by 22%, showing the beneficial effects exercise has on insulin effectiveness even in the absence of a post workout meal. The 'Immediately Post exercise' group increased insulin effectiveness by a whopping 44%, and in the 'delay' group it was improved by 19%. So a bout of exercise followed immediately with food increases insulin action, making this time the best to eat our high glycaemic carbs as it means our body will cope with the insulin much better. They also showed that more of the food was being used to restore muscle glycogen – showing potential food partitioning effects that would be beneficial to our body composition.

Folch et al (2001) tested the effects of a very large carbohydrate meal on subjects who had exercised. They found that fat burning continued with the group that had exercised and then eaten the biggest carbohydrate meal. They concluded that fat storing was totally suppressed following exercise, even when a massive meal is eaten. Where did the food go if it wasn't stored as fat? They found that the muscles had a greater store of glycogen; essentially the meal was diverted to the muscles as opposed to the fat stores. Although this study was to primarily look at the difference between low and high intensity exercise, it has implications for the optimal timing of our biggest meal.

Think of it this way – if two people both work out at around 4pm and person one eats a massive breakfast, getting almost all of their daily carbohydrates here, then after working out they eat nothing. The second person has only a small breakfast, small lunch, then after working out, they eat the biggest bulk of their daily carbohydrates and calories. Which person is going to get better nutrient storage? Obviously, as person two gets more nutrition after working out, they are going to improve their partitioning in favour of replenishing muscle stores (both protein and carbohydrate). Person one will have increased their amount of fat stores during their big breakfast, and will be left with an unfilled hole in their muscle stores as they didn't eat after exercising.

While it is true that this hole will be filled the next time they do eat, with our regimen of one day high calories followed by one day low, it may be 48 hours before they get enough nutrition to replenish the muscles fully, by which time the levels of beneficial hormones, insulin action and replenishment rates have dropped back down again.

24 hour nutrition

The main take-away points regarding nutrient timing are that, although what we eat after a workout may not have dramatic effects on our end body composition goals, they still matter. However, rather than obsessing over hour-by-hour meal timing, think of it more as a 24 hour window of opportunity.

If possible, the majority of your nutrition should come after your workout, as it will help with replenishing and restoring what was lost during your workout. Regarding protein, either get some during your pre-workout meal or post workout meal. Protein uptake in the muscle is much higher after exercise; Gianni et al (1997),

Koopman et al (2005), Miller et al (2003) all show increased muscle protein synthesis after exercise. So neglecting protein intake after your workout might be a bad idea. However, as long as you are getting adequate protein intake around your workout and in the 24-36 hours after your workout, this will be sufficient. As The Flexible Diet includes higher protein intake, we will be able to cover this with no problem. Even our low calorie days will have adequate protein amounts.

Regarding Carbohydrate intake – eating the majority of your carbs in the 24 hours after your workout will possibly create a preference to store those carbohydrates into muscles. Eating carbs immediately post workout may also help to improve insulin action and lower the amount of insulin your body produces (potentially a help for those worried about insulin levels). However, all of this information should not preside over flexibility and personal preference.

Chapter Summary

How many meals you have per day is not as important as what is contained in those meals. If you prefer to eat 1 big meal a day, or 7 smaller meals a day it is up to you. It will make no difference to your weight loss goals if the energy amount and composition of the diet is the same – as the science shows.

Eating more of your food earlier in the morning or later at night is of equal unimportance. Choose what suits you best and fits in with your lifestyle. The science is clear; it doesn't matter regarding weight loss or body composition.

Reducing meal frequency can help in cutting out daily caloric amounts. While it is generally taboo to say so, meal skipping can create a nice dent in your daily energy intake. The science shows that it will not negatively affect metabolism (more science shows it will actually increase metabolic rate in the short term).

For the less extreme, simply reducing the size of one or two of your meals can allow you the same benefits as meal skipping/meal frequency reduction without having to give up one of your meals. Replacing a meal with a protein shake or low energy density but high bulk food sources (fruit, veg, leafy greens etc.) can help to make the most of that reduced calorie meal.

By meal reduction or replacement, we can also use those reduced calories to shift them preferentially. For example, if you prefer to eat more food at night, eat less throughout the day so that you can have more calories at night. Or vice versa – if you prefer a lighter evening meal, eat more during the day and have a reduced calorie meal at night.

We could even use this caloric shifting to have more calories post-workout, when our body is set up for preferential storage of fuel, and our body may need more protein. Although, think of this in terms of 24 hour scales, not hour by hour minutiae.

Chapter 8
When Not to Eat

Several years ago, while working in Austria, I stumbled upon the idea of fasting after someone explained the magical benefits of it to me. I quickly disregarded it as hocus pocus – after all, everything I had ever learned about nutrition was purporting the opposite philosophy.

However, that night I went home and decided to take a look at some of the science to back up my opinion. What I found shocked me – all of the science I unearthed seemed to be counter to my original thinking. I saw study after study showing benefits to health, weight loss, longevity etc. How could this be?

This is probably the most controversial subject in the book; be warned that this idea is not for everyone, and you don't have to include it. However, with that disclaimer in place, it should be mentioned that you should not disregard the information in this chapter, as I did initially. It would be all too easy to not even entertain the idea of using the information presented to you in the next few pages. However, it would be more beneficial if you attempt this idea, as you could find it is a massive help in your goal to achieve your lower weight. So what is this idea? Welcome to the world of fasting.

Fasting is where you have a prolonged period without food. We all fast to a certain extent; every time we go to sleep we are going without food for a long time. That is why our first meal of the day is called breakfast, because you are breaking your fast. Traditionally, fasting is concerned with extending that time without food for 16, 24, 48 hours or even longer. Through reading this chapter we are going to learn what happens when we fast for extended periods of time, how we can use this information to improve our weight loss and how to implement it into our lives. We will also look at some of the other health benefits that fasting offers that can extend far beyond weight-loss.

Who Fasts?

Fasting has been part of religious practices for many years. Muslims practice fasting during Ramadan; a whole 30 days without eating, drinking and smoking between dawn and dusk. This means periods of 16-18 hours or so without food. Buddhist Monks and nuns refrain from eating after their noon meal, resulting in an afternoon 'til dawn 'eating break' of around 18 hours or so.

Fasting also litters the literature of Christianity, with the day of atonement being a full day fast once per year, with further examples of Moses, David and Joel participating in this act. Roman Catholics also see several calendar days per year of fasting or partial fasts. Hindu's, Mormons, Jews, Sikhs, and many other religions also practice partial or full fasts as part of their faith. In many cases it is a character test, a strength of will and devotion to their God(s), or a nudge down the road to self mastery and enlightenment.

What Happens When We Fast?

Most people think that, if we go for too long without food, our blood sugar levels drop dangerously low. However, in healthy human subjects, our blood sugar levels are maintained in a very tight range. When we have gone without food for a long time, our body releases glucagon, which helps to convert our stored glucose into sugar - the end result being our blood sugar levels are normalized. Only in a person who is hypoglycaemic does this not happen, and these people are few and far between.

When all the carbohydrates in our blood have been used up and our liver glycogen is approaching depletion, our body increases the rate of fat burning, and we go into a state of Ketosis (where our body uses ketones from fat to power itself) if the fast is overly prolonged. Growth hormone is released which helps mobilize our stored fat, and insulin levels drop so that our body is more efficient at this task. Literally, less fat is stored and more is used to power our body and metabolism.

Metabolic Rate

As we have already seen in our last chapter, during a fasting session of up to 72 hours (3 days), our metabolic rate actually increases slightly. This is why it is not metabolically detrimental if we skip one meal. Benedict et al (1919), Mansell (1990), Webber (1994) and Zauner (2000) all found increases in metabolic rate during fasts of between 12 and 72 hours. This increase in metabolic rate during short term fasting is due to the energy costs of gluconeogenesis (your body creating its own sugar), ketogenesis and fatty acid recycling.

If we also remember the study by Heilbronn et al (2005), where subjects who did a full fast (no food) every other day did not see a drop in metabolic rate for 21 days. Their body also switched to a huge increase in fat burning over this period. This maintenance of metabolic rate occurred in spite of the 2.5% loss in body weight and 4% loss of fat mass; showing an overall caloric deficit. This is a relatively extreme amount of fasting - essentially half of the week without eating anything for 3 whole weeks. Also, it was in an alternating fashion, which mimics our calorie cycling that we are doing. But instead of cycling between high and low calories, the subjects were cycling between high and *no* calories. It is worth mentioning that, during the study, people had higher levels of hunger than normal. However, we can eliminate this by not fasting as extremely. For example, fasting one day a week would not produce the same negative effects on hunger as fasting every other day.

Fasting is Difficult

Many people will be reading most of this, seeing the potential benefits and wishing they had the ability to do it. These people will also imagine fasting to be incredibly difficult and they would never be able to do it. However, before you skip to the next section of the book, entertain the idea that fasting is not as difficult as you would imagine. Many people report it actually being very liberating the first time they do it. I certainly didn't think I had the ability to do it the first time I heard about it, but I decided to attempt it and found it incredibly manageable.

We also have many options when it comes to fasting. It doesn't have to be (and I wouldn't start out with) a whole day of fasting. We could start with a smaller version and build up as we become more tolerant and understanding of how we personally respond to fasting. I started with a 16 hour fast, simply by skipping breakfast one day, and worked my way up to a full 24 hour and even (eventually) a 72 hour fast.

It certainly trained me to not be as dependent upon food as I believed I was. It is quite freeing to know that you can (should it be necessary) survive quite comfortably without your regular meal pattern. Certainly, in the wild we wouldn't have had the luxury of steady meals. We have almost certainly evolved with a more 'feast and famine' approach to eating, so our bodies are perfectly capable of managing it. Even more-so (as we will find out), our bodies may just thrive on an occasional fast.

Fasting and Weight Loss

People reading the first few paragraphs about what happens when we fast are undoubtedly thinking that the major benefit to fasting would be increased fat loss. While this is true during the fast, we still have to see the bigger picture. Burning a lot of fat while fasting gives us no advantage if we are to make up for it when we break the fast. For example, if fasting for one day a week allows you to cut out an extra 2500 calories then it will cause more fat loss than if you hadn't fasted. However, if you are to fast one day and then eat double the calories the next day, the net effects on fat stores would be the same (although there are several studies to show this eating pattern could still offer other health benefits).

The Heilbronn Study found that by fasting on alternate days (and feeding as much as they wanted to on non-fasting days), subjects lost 4% body-fat in 22 days. Varady et al. (2011) also looked at an alternate day modified fast, where subjects ate as normal one day, then ate only 25% of maintenance calories the next. After 8 weeks, subjects lost 5.6 KG (12-13 lb), as well as experiencing other health benefits. Johnson et al (2007) did a similar protocol for 8 weeks, where subjects alternated between eating as they wished and days of only 20% of maintenance calories. During the trial, the subjects lost 8% of their initial weight.

More recently, Harvie et al (2011) found that people placed on a 6 month diet of alternate day calorie restriction (25% calories one day, eat what you want the next) versus a more constant caloric restriction lost the same amount of weight. In 2013, Eshghinia and Mohammadzadeh found alternate day fasting to create a 6KG (13lb) weight loss in 8 weeks – again adding to the vast bulk of data out there showing the benefits of fasting to weight loss.

Fasting works in the same way that caloric restriction works – by cutting down the amount of energy coming in. For those reasons, fasting is not particularly magical, although it can certainly be an extra option to you when creating your Flexible Diet. However, on top of weight loss benefits, there could be some other potential health benefits, as we will now explore.

What is the most extreme form of fasting has been conducted in science? In 1973, Stewart and Fleming had a 27 year old male fasting under medical supervision for a whopping 382 days. While he lost 276lb during that time, he felt no ill effects.

Benefits to Health

Animal studies

Carlson and Hoelzel (1946) were one of the first to look into fasting in rats. They found they could increase the lifespan of rats by 20% by putting them on a regimen of one day fasting, and 2 days eating what they wanted. Honjoh et al (2009) found that by putting C Elegans worms on an alternate day fast, they could extend their lifespan by 40%. Katare et al (2009) found that intermittent fasting improved the survival rate of rats following chronic heart failure. Halagappa et al (2007) saw improvements in mouse models of Alzheimer's disease. More impressively, Anson Et al (2003) reported that when mice were kept on an alternate day fast, they experienced health benefits above pure caloric restriction, including reduced blood glucose levels, insulin levels, and resistance to brain injury.

Mattson (2000) found that both caloric restriction and alternate day fasting has positive effects on experimental models of Alzheimer's, Parkinson's, Huntington's disease and stroke. They give an explanation for how it works, but it is far too complicated for this book, although if you are interested in further reading, the references are in the back of the book. Mattson also states that this type of dietary manipulation can improve the brain's capacity for plasticity and repair, potentially leading to improvements in learning and memory. This makes sense evolutionary; if food is relatively scarce, it is of a higher value to have a better mental capacity. The hunter who could learn faster and remember where food sources are during times of scarcity would be more likely to survive. Duan et al (2003) also confirmed the Huntington's disease retardation, life extending and glucose normalizing effects of intermittent fasting on mice. There is also evidence from research by Siegel et al (1988), Descamps et al (2005) and Hsieh et al (2005) that alternate day fasting shows anti cancer effects, although this needs to be thoroughly researched.

Human studies

There are no long term studies on the effects of fasting and feasting on humans, mainly due to the ethical and procedural complications involved with creating such a study. However, in 2007, Johnson et al found that Asthmatics placed on an alternate day fasting protocol not only lost 8% of their weight, but mood and energy elevated, total cholesterol decreased, markers of inflammation improved and oxidative stress improved. Also, their symptoms of asthma improved greatly.

In the Spanish medical records in 1957, elderly subjects over the age of 65 were put on an alternate day partial fasting of either 56% or 144% of their daily caloric needs. Their weight was maintained during the study, as caloric input/output was balanced. It was found that more people in the normal diet died than in the fasting protocol (13 out of 60 compared with 6 out of 60). Although these results are not statistically significant, the alternate day fasting subjects spent only 123 days in hospital compared with 219 days from the normal control diet – very significant results.

Research from the Intermountain Medical Center Heart Institute reported in 2011 that periodic fasting is good for your heart and your health. They found that fasting lowers your risk of coronary artery disease (CAD) by lowering blood cholesterol, insulin resistance and hence risk of diabetes. Bhutani et al (2010) found after 10 weeks of alternate day fasting, bodyweight and waist circumference were reduced, fat mass decreased (although lean body mass was retained fully), bad cholesterol was reduced, good cholesterol was maintained; great news for our health. In the Varady et al study (2009), Coronary Artery Disease risks were also improved; blood pressure decreased, bad cholesterol decreased, and good cholesterol remained unchanged. Heilbronn's 2005 study not only showed weight loss, but a decrease in fasting insulin levels. There have been suggestions from Roth et al (2002) that lowered levels of fasting insulin is associated with longer life in humans. An added bonus of this style of eating was that the subjects did not see significant decreases in their resting metabolic rate, despite the drop in body mass.

While most of the studies looked at doing a 24 hour fast (or partial fast) followed by a 24 hour feast, it is expected that a daily/every other day fast of 14-20 hours or so would produce similar health benefits. Indeed, the studies that included a small amount of calories on the 'fasting days' still showed the same benefits, so this is likely the case. Halberg et al (2005) looked into this exact protocol, placing subjects on a 20 hour fast once every 2 days. While subjects maintained their weight (showing caloric balance), insulin action was greatly improved, showing signs of decreased diabetes risk. This shows us that the **beneficial health effects may persist even without any weight loss**.

Most of the studies show short term health benefits with this type of eating pattern. The lack of long term studies means that we cannot jump to wild conclusions just yet, but the research does seem promising. The only long term results we can analyse are the people who practice these regimens during the course of their lifetime.

Types of Fasting

There are three main types of fasting we will look at which can fit into our Flexible Diet. These are the one day fast, the partial fast, and intermittent fasting.

One Day Fast

While probably the more daunting version of fasting, a one day fast is a great way to make a large deficit in our weekly/daily caloric intake. As an example, we have a person who needs 2500 calories per day to maintain their weight. This person eats their 2500 calories a day for 6 days, and then completely fasts for one whole day. That means they have created a 2500 calorie weekly deficit, equivalent to around half a pound of weight loss (typically). If this person did this complete fast twice weekly, they would create a 5000 calorie deficit.

It is not recommended to do a complete fast three times a week, as the study by Heilbronn (2005) showed that hunger remains elevated when fasting is done too often. However, once a week is fine, or twice a week is also manageable if separated by a few maintenance or high calorie days.

The main benefit to this way of fasting is mental, but it also has several physical advantages. Mentally, going without food for only 24 hours can be very manageable. It can be a lot less painful than you would imagine, and much less excruciating than the same deficit over the course of the week. For example, making a 400 calorie deficit a day, every day, is much more arduous for most people than just going 24 hours without food once a week. The rest of the time you get to eat as normal, it is just one day of hunger rather than 7. You will probably find that the hunger will not be as severe as you thought. It is almost like ripping off a plaster, we get it out of the way so we can carry on as normal. Why not start the week with a full day fast when your motivation is high, and then the rest of the week you can eat as normal, or cycle your calories as before.

Don't forget, if you go a full day without food, this may technically be 36 or more hours of fasting. If the last meal you eat is at 8pm on a Sunday night, then you fast all of Monday before eating a breakfast on Tuesday at 8am – that is 36 hours.

The Partial Fast

This is similar to many of the protocols used in the studies we looked at. This is a less extreme form of fasting than the full day fast. Basically, using this protocol, you will dramatically reduce your calories during one day. For example, you may only consume 20-50% of your normal Daily calories during that day, cutting down from 2000 (for example) to just 500-1000 calories.

This will require a lot less willpower than the full day fasting, and it may be a nice way to introduce the idea of fasting into your life. You can spread those calories as you desire, perhaps in two smaller meals through the day, or one much larger meal at one point in the day. Be sure to make those calories go as far as possible

– 500 calories of vegetables is much more filling than 500 calories of chocolate.

Intermittent fasting

Another way to incorporate fasting into your diet is to do shorter daily fasts. Rather than going for 24 hours without food, try doing a 14, 16 or even 20 hour fast. For example, you could have your last meal at 9pm the night before, and then have your first meal of the day at 1pm the following day, resulting in a 16 hour fast. Basically, this is the same as skipping breakfast and having your normal lunch and dinner. This is much easier to manage than a full day fast, as you only have to skip one meal.

If you just can't go without breakfast, the other way that you could work this is to eat your last meal at 6pm, then have your breakfast the following morning at 8am resulting in a 14 hour fast, although this tends to be less workable as people like to go out for dinner and social occasions, whereas not eating breakfast usually encounters fewer problems.

This protocol may sound very similar to the partial fast, but during intermittent fasting you are not necessarily reducing the calories below normal. In fact, you could do intermittent fasting in conjunction with your higher calorie days if you wanted to. For example, you may skip breakfast, before having a much bigger lunch and dinner equalling 100% of your normal daily calories. This is essentially shifting calories around to where you desire.

A one-meal-a-day pattern could also work with this. It would essentially be classed as a 24 hour fast, where you eat your only meal of the day, and then it is 24 hours until you eat again. If workable, this means you can eat really huge and satiating meals while still dieting. Lots of people find it very satisfying to eat 1700 calories of food in one sitting while still losing weight. It certainly isn't for everyone, but it is an option.

Not so Fast

So how should we go about implementing fasting into our diets? Some people will want to jump straight into it and try a full fast straight away. While this is possible, it is not recommended, as your body will not currently be used to 24 hours without food. We have grown so accustomed to having whatever sustenance we wish at our fingertips, that our body may have never been through more than 12 hours without food in our life.

However, we can build up our ability to fast, and at the same time we can check our current tolerance. While you are fasting, it is highly recommended to remain well-hydrated. Water is the beverage of choice, as it is calorie free and hence will not spoil your fast. However, tea and coffee can also be a suitable supplement, although don't load it with heavy milk and creamer or it will spoil the point of the fast. Be warned that caffeine containing beverages will have more potent effects if you are fasted, as there is no food in your gut to dilute the effects.

Also, make sure you consult your Doctor/Physician before undertaking any extreme regimen like this. You may not be in a condition to be able to do fasting, and it is beyond the scope of this book to look at it on an individual level. So make sure you get prior approval of your medical practitioner.

If you would like to include a 24 hour fast in your weekly regimen, I would suggest starting with just skipping breakfast at first. Go one day where you eliminate this meal, and see how you feel – or even simply reduce the size of your breakfast. If your last meal was 8pm the previous night and you eat lunch at 1pm, this is a 17 hour fast. Eat your lunch and dinner as normal, making sure that they are the same size that you would normally have. Repeat this on a few separate occasions, making sure that you do not do it twice in a row. A good way to introduce this would be on your low calorie days, as it is the easiest way to reduce calories.

The first few times you try this, you may find that you are very hungry during the fasting stage. This is temporary and will pass after 30 minutes or so, your body has been trained to release hunger inducing hormones at these times, but you will get over it as it doesn't last long.

As your body starts becoming accustomed to breakfast skipping, try to prolong the time that you break the fast - eating lunch later in the day, for example. You could also work in a reverse fashion, eating your last meal of the previous day a few hours earlier. When you feel fully confident that you can achieve it, try a full 24 hour fast. If you eat your last meal at 8pm the night before, you would essentially break your fast at 8pm the following day. This is a great test of willpower and discipline, and you may be surprised at how much easier it is to achieve than you think. Try to limit the calories in your first meal after your fast, as they will be counted towards your daily total. So although this method will not cut out a full day worth of calories, it can make a large deficit in your daily/weekly calorie total.

Make sure that you do not do this type of fasting too many times during a week. I would start with one session a week until you feel you can cope, and maybe go to 2 sessions a week, although split them apart with high calorie days. Heilbronn showed that 24 hour fasting can be successfully completed every other day, however, the effects on hunger levels never seemed to go away. By limiting yourself to 2 x 24 hour fasts per week it should not be a problem, but only you will be able to evaluate.

Nutrient Timing and Fasting

In the last chapter, we looked at the effects exercise has on our need for certain nutrient intake. Obviously, fasting will have an effect on this. If we are exercising and then fasting straight after, this may not be the most optimal way of creating our desired body composition.

As a result, I would recommend fasting on non-exercise days, and try to keep the fasting times as far away from when you have exercised as possible. Below are some examples to help you figure out when to do fasting, depending upon when you personally prefer to exercise.

Intermittent fasting, Morning exerciser

For a morning exerciser who finishes their workout at 8am (for example), we would exercise and follow this up with a 4-10 hour eating window. The last meal of the day would be at 12-6pm resulting in a 14-20 hour fasting period. This would give your body enough nutrition, and if your last meal of the day is the largest, it should still be fuelling you for the majority of the fast.

This type of eating could be potentially troublesome, only in terms of social behaviour. To have your last meal at midday means you would have to miss out on dinner with family and friends. This is obviously not ideal, also for the fact that you would have to eat all of your calories during the morning. With work and other duties, this can also prove inconvenient. However, another way of doing this would be to include fasting only on your low calorie, non-exercise days. During your exercise days, you would eat a normal diet after your workout, but non exercise days would include a fast starting from 12-6pm until next morning. This means that you would only have to skip certain dinners, allowing you to schedule days where you will exercise around days where you will be going out for meals.

Intermittent Fasting, Midday exerciser

For a midday exerciser, things can be a little easier. You would skip your breakfast, and then break your fast before your workout (with a glass of milk or small protein shake if you didn't want to workout in a fasted state). After exercising, you would have a 4-10 hour window where you eat all of your allotted calories.

This is probably the easiest of all the protocols to deal with, as skipping breakfast is usually not a problem for most people both physically and mentally. It also allows you to go to later night social functions and have dinner with the family every night. This type of fasting protocol can be maintained every single day, as it doesn't disturb the normal flow of everyday life, unless early morning breakfasting is part of your life. You could, alternatively, limit your partial fasting days to your low calorie days. This would allow you to eat breakfast on your workout days if you wished to. As your workout days contain more calories, it can easily allow breakfast while maintaining high levels of post-workout nutrition.

If you are like myself, I prefer to fast throughout the day and then eat all my calories after my workout, resulting in huge 'post-workout' meals that get shuttled into repairing lean body mass – which brings us to our next version.

Intermittent Fasting, Evening exerciser

Someone who finishes exercising around 7pm could choose to fast completely until their pre-workout meal (glass of milk or protein shake). After working out, they could then have a 4-6 hour feeding window where they eat the majority of their daily calories. For people who like to eat big and don't mind eating late, this can be a very workable option. However, with workout days being our high calorie days, we are often consuming huge amounts of food in this small window. While studies have shown that this is not a problem, for some it can cause digestive discomfort and poor sleep. You would have to decide for yourself if this is a good option or not. Some people see the opposite effects and fall asleep like a baby after their big meal. But for other 'after work exercisers' who do not like this set-up, there are more options.

You could break your fast at lunch-time, or a little later in the day. Then have your 6-10 hour eating window, within which you would exercise. An example of this would be someone who eats their lunch at 3pm (usually not the biggest meal), finishes exercising at 7pm and follows it with their biggest meal of the day. This would be an example of a 4 hour eating window. However, someone could also add another meal later in the evening, extending the feeding period to 6-8 hours (depending on how late the last meal is). This can be a great set-up for your diet, allowing a 16-20 hour fast along with hugely satiating post workout meals.

Full day fasting/partial fasting and exercise

The main issue we have here is if we conduct a full day of fasting or dramatically reduced food intake straight after exercise. As this is the time when our body needs nutrients the most (especially protein), it could hamper our attempts to minimize muscle loss during the dieting process. However, there are ways around this.

If you limit your full fasting days to ones which don't coincide with your exercise days, this shouldn't be a problem. Doing your full day fast on Monday, then eating as normal and working out from Tuesday onwards will not interfere.

This is one of the reasons I would guard against doing full day or partial fasts too many times in a week, as it is tough to organize your nutrition and workouts. However, there is a possible scenario where it would work nicely. If you were to workout in the morning, follow it up with eating as normal for the rest of the day, then do a full or partial fast the following day, you will still get enough post workout nutrition.

Flexibility

So, as you can see, there is a method for everyone. Whether you choose to do partial daily fasts every other day, intermittently, or whether you prefer to dive right in and fast completely for a day, there is an option to suit you. It is not a case of 'more is better'; as with everything in life, we need to be sensible about these things. But utilizing fasting can easily help us with the other areas we are looking to include, such as calorie control and calorie cycling. Try different options and see which one sits best with you, which one fits in best with your lifestyle, eating habits and exercising preferences.

Don't forget, this is just an option. You don't have to do it at all!

Chapter Summary

Fasting has been shown to provide not only impressive weight loss, but many health benefits, even when calories are maintained.

Improvements to insulin sensitivity, diabetes risk, cholesterol, cardiovascular disease, Cancer, Parkinsons, and potential life extending benefits are all hypothesized, with evidence supporting. Also, inflammatory illnesses such as asthma and arthritis are helped with fasting.

There are many options for fasting, from intermittent daily fasts, a partial fast or a full blown 1-2 day fast.

Try first by eating a smaller breakfast than normal, or extending the time until you have breakfast (or skip it altogether).

Extend that period further until you can do a 20 hour fast. Why not try and do a 24 hour fast where you eat one meal in the day, 24 hours after your last meal. This could be a reduced calorie meal (as in a partial fast), or you could eat all of your allotted calories in this meal (as in intermittent fasting).

If you feel comfortable and able, attempt a full day fast.

Fasting can help us to re-distribute calories around in our day or even week, so that we can eat more around workout days etc. or at times where we desire.

Chapter 9
Examples

Now that we have the theory and the main points behind The Flexible Diet, we can start to put it all together into a workable plan. In order to help, this chapter is dedicated to looking at some simple example plans. Essentially, the possibilities are endless, and while you could copy these plans directly, they are there mainly to help you understand further how you could put this information into your own life. I want you to take control of the process and invent your own version of the diet. If you are going to use these plans, you will need to adjust the caloric amounts to suit you personally.

Make sure to be adaptable with this process. The whole premise behind The Flexible Diet is that it is yours to own and it is flexible – hence the name. If you decide on one protocol and it doesn't fit your life one day, feel free to change it. For example, say you are normally a big-lunch eater and you have an important work dinner coming up where you know you will be consuming more than normal, flip it. Eat less for lunch, so you can shuffle those daily calories around. I recommend occasionally switching the diet up in design to keep it fresher and keep your motivation high – and you also may stumble upon one which really clicks with you.

Sample days

Some people will prefer a nibbling pattern, some people may prefer a gorging pattern. Some people will prefer to eat most food at night, some prefer a lighter dinner but a heavier breakfast and lunch to get them through the day. Below are some examples of 2 day plans you can emulate/test out, alongside how they might fit in with exercise days. Each plan is for a person averaging 1800 calories per day (perhaps they have a maintenance of 2300 calories).

6 meals a day pattern

Time	Workout day	Rest day
8AM	300 calories	300 calories
10AM	300 calories	
12PM	300 calories	300 calories
2PM	300 calories	300 calories
4PM	EXERCISE	300 calories
6PM	600 calories	
8PM	300 calories	300 calories

This example is much more of a nibbling pattern which **averages** 1800 calories per day at 300 calories per meal. 300 calories can be quite a lot of food if you pack it with nutritious, low energy dense sources. This pattern would allow a nice size post-workout meal also. The exercise time could also move around when you desire and it wouldn't affect the diet at all.

But you don't have t eat as frequently or have the same sized meals each time, as we will see in our next example.

3 meals a day pattern

Time	Workout day	Rest day
8AM	300 calories	300 calories
1PM	500 calories	500 calories
5PM	EXERCISE	
7PM	1200 calories	800 calories

This example shows a much less frequent but much larger meal size (which can be a lot more satiating). The post workout meal could potentially be massive, or you could spread the calories around a lot more evenly if you preferred. Again, this meal plan averages 1800 calories per day.

2 meals a day pattern

Time	Workout day	Rest day
8AM	1000 calories	800 calories
5PM	EXERCISE	
7PM	1000 calories	800 calories

This pattern may suit someone who likes to have a big breakfast which can sustain them throughout the day, before finishing with a big dinner.

Morning intermittent fasting

This below plan is very similar to the last one, but instead of skipping lunch, this plan skips breakfast. Essentially, this is intermittent fasting, as there would be a period of 17 hours between the last meal and the next one.

Time	Workout day	Rest day
8AM		
12	800 calories	800 calories
5PM	EXERCISE	
7PM	1200 calories	800 calories

Again, this suits the person who likes to eat larger meals, as they can pack a bigger energy density into the smaller meal frequency. This pattern also provides a lot of post-workout nutrition, and may suit an afternoon or evening exerciser.

Morning exerciser (and intermittent fasting)

Perhaps you like to exercise in the morning and would still like to try intermittent fasting. This may be a good version for you.

Time	Workout day	Rest day
7AM	EXERCISE	
8AM	800 Calories	600 calories
2PM	1200 calories	1000 calories

This would give your body a nice big meal before you go into the fast, and can be perfect for someone who never feels hungry at night. This meal pattern is not for everyone, as very few people like to miss dinner - so below is another option for a morning exerciser.

Morning Exerciser 2

Time	Workout day	Rest day
7AM	EXERCISE	
8AM	500 calories	400 calories
2PM	800 calories	600 calories
8PM	700 calories	600 calories

Again, as with all of the plans, this supplies an average of 1800 calories a day, with 2000 calories on exercise days and 1600 on rest days.

Some people may prefer to cycle their calories a bit more wildly in order to take advantage of days where they can really fill up on food. Below is an example of the same average caloric amount (1800/day), but with a more unbalanced distribution.

Feast and Famine

Time	Workout day	Rest day
8AM	400 calories	300 calories
1PM	800 calories	300 calories
5PM	EXERCISE	
7PM	1100 calories	700 calories

This method spreads the calories to 2300 on exercise days and only 1300 on rest days. This is a little more extreme, but can be nicely manageable for many people. It may also be a nice option if you know you are going to be eating a lot one day, you can simply lower the calories of the next day.

Weekly Plans

On top of our daily plans, we can plan the week in more flexible ways to accommodate individual preference. Here, we will look at some of the possible weekly plans so you get an idea of where you would like to go with your own Flexible Diet.

The Three Day Diet

This is an example of a week where you are essentially dieting only 3 days in the week, as the other days are higher calorie days.

Day	Calories	Exercise
Monday	2000	Yes
Tuesday	1600	
Wednesday	2000	Yes
Thursday	1600	
Friday	2000	Yes
Saturday	2000	
Sunday	1600	

In this example, both Friday and Saturday are higher calorie days, as those are usually the days which we are out having meals with friends/at social occasions etc. For a person with a maintenance caloric intake of 2300 per day, this would provide roughly a 3300 calorie weekly deficit.

The Two Day Diet

Perhaps you prefer to rip the plaster off and get your dieting done in two days so you can go back to eating normally? If so, we could use partial fasting as a way of accomplishing this.

Day	Calories	Exercise
Monday	500	
Tuesday	2300	Yes
Wednesday	2300	
Thursday	500	
Friday	2300	Yes
Saturday	2300	
Sunday	2300	

In this example, the dieting is essentially done only on Monday and Thursday, and timed so that they don't coincide with exercise days or 24 hours post exercise (to ensure adequate recovery nutrition).

This pattern still provides a weekly deficit of 3600 calories due to the partial fasting days, even though the other 5 days are eating at a maintenance level and essentially not dieting. This should provide a slow and stable but sustainable weight loss weekly.

The Five Day diet

Some people would rather diet during the week when they are working, but live a more normal life on the weekends.

Day	Calories	Exercise
Monday	1800	Yes
Tuesday	1600	
Wednesday	1800	Yes
Thursday	1600	
Friday	1800	Yes
Saturday	2300	
Sunday	2300	

For a person with a 2300 calorie maintenance, this would create roughly a 2900 calorie weekly deficit, while still allowing you to enjoy your weekends a bit more. Be warned, it is easy to blow your entire week's effort by carelessly gorging on the weekend – so keep track and don't go overboard.

Feast and famine

Some people may prefer to have a diet which looks more like the alternate day fasting protocols. This intersperses days of greatly reduced caloric intake with days of much higher intake.

Day	Calories	Exercise
Monday	1200	
Tuesday	2400	Yes
Wednesday	1200	
Thursday	2400	Yes
Friday	1200	
Saturday	2400	Yes
Sunday	2000	

On exercise days, this would mean a much higher calorie intake. Ideally, most of those calories would come after the workout, so this may involve an afternoon workout and large afternoon and evening meals. For a person with a maintenance of 2300 calories per day, this protocol provides a weekly deficit of 3300 calories, even though some days actually go slightly above maintenance.

A Bit of Everything

Some people may decide to do a little bit of everything, as shown.

Day	Calories	Exercise
Monday	2400	Yes
Tuesday	1600	
Wednesday	500	
Thursday	2000	Yes
Friday	1600	
Saturday	2300	
Sunday	0	

This plan would provide a 5700 calorie weekly deficit, and includes a full day fast, a partial fast (Wednesday), and 3 higher calorie days close to workout days.

Chapter 10

Flexibility

Hopefully, through reading the main principles of this diet, you can see how to create a plan that allows you the best of all worlds. The main principle, or 'golden rule' if you wish, is calorie control. Without this, the diet is doomed for failure. But abiding by this principle means you can eat what you want and still lose weight. No foods are off limits with this diet, so long as the daily caloric needs are, on average, not exceeded.

You need to be aware of how many calories you need to maintain your weight, and you must eat below this level if you wish to lose weight. We can use several methods to measure the amount of energy we intake, but the best way is to count calories at the back of the packets, or by weighing the food you eat and using online calorie counters - at least until you are able to give a good estimate naturally. It is not important to be obsessive about it, but if you are not losing weight then you are clearly eating too much and must find a way to reduce calories.

The main problem with a reduction in calories is the persistent hunger we experience with it. This is effectively counteracted by cycling your calories between high and low periods every day, if possible. As long as the calories eaten at the end of the week are less than what has been burned, your body will be in a dieting state. This is effective due to the fact you are essentially dieting only half of the time. It is much easier to go through the hunger, as you know that tomorrow is a normal calorie day, or even slightly higher than usual. This kind of physical and mental relief is missing from almost every other diet.

Our other goal during the diet is to preserve as much lean body mass as possible. This is helped through the use of calorie cycling, exercise, increased protein consumption and nutrient timing. By exercising, we are stimulating our body to hold on to as much lean body mass throughout the diet, or even create a more solid, toned/athletic physique. Combining this with increased protein and more food after your workout, we are creating a plan that turns your body into what you have always dreamed of, but never thought possible. Maintaining lean body mass will help you speed up your weight loss goals by avoiding plateaus, maintaining/improving metabolism, and making sure that more of the weight loss comes from your fat stores. It is also going to help you maintain your new physique when you have achieved where you are happy.

Mentally, the principles that make up this diet make it superior to any other. A successful diet by nature is one that you can stick to for enough time to see results. Through the use of calorie cycling and fasting, we are able to have days involving very large satiating meals. Adding extra protein to your diet 'supercharges' the long term satiety, leaving you less hungry than other diets.

With this diet, you are not changing the foods you eat; you are still able to eat your favourite foods whether they are deemed good or bad for you. This means that you never have to 'come off' the diet, as you were never really on one in the first place. Most diets that are limiting your food choice are set up to fail because when you come off it, you end up gorging on all the foods that you missed out on, leaving you with deep rooted subconscious mechanisms that prevent us going on another diet.

Lastly, through fasting we can see that we have many more flexible options available to us when it comes to planning our meal frequency, and hence meal size. Less frequent meals equal bigger meals. We can also use fasting or partial fasting to cut out a big chunk of weekly calories when we are feeling motivated enough to do so.

By lowering our overall calorie intake through the act of dieting, we are losing fat mass and hence improving our health in many respects. Through the tactics employed to preserve lean body mass, we are improving our insulin sensitivity and further decreasing our fat mass. Fasting is yet another strategy, as improved insulin sensitivity results from prolonged periods without foods. Add this to the other beneficial effects seen when weight is lowered and exercise is introduced, along with improved nutritional quality of our foods, and we have a winning formula for success in health.

Fitting it Into Your Life

Everybody is busy. People are too busy to start a diet, too busy to continue it when they have started, and too busy to re-start when they have failed. There is always going to be something that comes up when you are dieting, something that could potentially ruin your success. But it doesn't have to. Life happens, but there are always ways around these problems.

With The Flexible Diet, there are no more excuses for complete slip ups, as they can easily fit into the regimen unnoticed. You can effortlessly work around social functions, upcoming meals, all you can eat food competitions etc. without ruining your goals. The worst thing to see is someone constantly starting a new diet as their previous one failed from a small error. They slipped up a little one evening, and then decided they would start again next week. This person then 'forgets' to start again next week, ending up starting all over again in 3 months time, 5 pounds heavier than when they first decided to go on a diet. If this sounds like you, then you should not fret anymore as The Flexible Diet has come into your life.

Social Functions

If you know that you have a meal coming up one evening, for example, it does not have to be such a big problem. Firstly, we could take steps to make sure we fit our exercise session on this day (before you go out for your meal); this means that you will be on a high calorie day and it can easily fit into your daily total.

Great, but what if you can't exercise that day, for whatever reason? You could always do your exercise session the day before, even if it is your low calorie day. While not optimal, it can definitely serve as a useful back up plan. As long as after exercising you move most of your daily calories to post workout, you should have enough nutrition to keep the positive effects going. And besides, one day of poor post workout nutrition is not going to destroy everything. The small advantage you gain from effective post workout nutrition is seen after consistent application of the rule. One day of tinkering will, at worst, make an unnoticeable dent in your gains. However, stopping a diet completely will have profound effects on your overall success.

Why not also take advantage of our fasting rule? By including a partial fast or limiting calorie intake throughout the day, we can breeze through a social function and still lose weight. For example, you could decide to just graze on low energy-dense foods throughout the day (such as low calorie vegetables, soups or fruit etc.) and not really having a main meal, making sure that you save up chunk of your daily calories for the evening.

At the end of the day, as long as you haven't exceeded your daily limit, you will be fine. We could also use the same principle, but do a partial fast by eating nothing throughout the day, breaking our fast at lunch with a smaller than normal meal, or even forgoing lunch (if you have the ability) so that you can eat more freely during the event. Other options include a full 24 hour fast the day before, which could create a calorie debt which more than exceeds what you will eat in your event. Or you could also do a full 24 hour fast after the event - probably a better option, as your body will have more food being digested after the event, potentially making the 24 hour fast more comfortably completed.

There are still more tools available to us. Why not move calories around in our weekly plan? If your event is on Saturday night, try cutting 100 calories a day on all other days, allowing you to go over your normal allowance by 600 calories on the night and still maintain the same weekly calories. You could equally cut 200 calories from 3 other nights in the week, and have the same 600 calorie excess on Saturday.

There are so many combinations, decide what is best for you. Why not use all of the above tactics to a certain degree; move some calories around in the week to the day of the event, exercising before the event during the day, making sure it is a high calorie day in your weekly cycle, meal skipping before the event, and even include a full 24 hour fast the day after the event. With all of these tactics employed (or even just one or two), we can see that it is easy to include a social event without having to put the diet on hold or sabotage it completely. Most people see an event coming up and say that they can't begin/continue their diet now, as the event will ruin it; let this no longer be you. Besides, just because it is a social meal doesn't mean you have to go out and eat the entire restaurant. You could always choose a lighter option on the menu, or ask for your meal without certain sauces etc. I am the last person to tell someone not to enjoy their food, but you can always make more sensible choices when you are out. Wouldn't that be a novel idea.

Slip Ups Happen

If all else fails, allow a slip up. If we expect to be perfect during a diet, we are probably setting ourselves up for more failure than success. If you achieved a 500 calorie weekly deficit rather than your preferred 2000, it is still a step in the right direction, just a smaller one. Even if you make a big slip up (and with all our tactics in place, this should happen less often), so what! People who succeed in diets are usually more flexible about their approach, and see slip ups as a bump in the journey. If you go up one or two pounds in a week, it is not a disaster. Just get back on track and start again, learning from what went wrong.

Most of the time, fluctuations in water weight can easily account for 5 or more pounds of instant weight gain. This water weight will come right back off again when you resume the diet. But if you stop the diet in order to start again at a later date, your chances of success are slim to none. When we look at goal setting during the next chapter, we can see how to forecast for these blips, and still achieve huge goals. During the periodization section (upcoming) we can see how going to a maintenance week (where you do not lose weight, but stabilize it) can aid you in your goals. Maybe you could re-frame your 'slip up' as an unplanned maintenance week. There are just so many options, it seems so flexible!

The Maintenance Day

This is such a simple idea, but could be the biggest factor in the success of your diet and eventually achieving your goals. It's called "The Maintenance Day". So incredible yet so simple – disappointingly simple in fact. But adding this idea to your dieting arsenal will revolutionize your ability to keep on track.

The Maintenance Day is exactly what it says on the tin. While most people see dieting as an 'either-or' situation, where they are either dieting or eating everything in sight, we can throw in a middle-ground, more moderate approach. Why not have a day where we simply eat at maintenance calories? We are neither moving forwards nor backwards, but we are maintaining what we have achieved.

For example, if you are going along in your planned diet, you have lost a nice amount of weight and then, unexpectedly, a social function pops up, or you are having a day of poor motivation, or you simply want a day off – do a maintenance day. Rather than have this unexpected blip completely ruin your diet and then set off a chain reaction which derails you further, simply shift to maintenance calories for the day. You don't even have to workout on this day – take a day off.

This is much more 'big-picture' thinking. Rather than the goal being "I must be constantly moving forwards", it's ok to sometimes stand still. See it as a resting point before you push on forwards again. The Flexible Diet is supposed to be this way.

As we will see later, this can also transform into occasional 'Maintenance Weeks' where we have a whole week of standing still. What you have to understand, and this next line is very important, is that **maintaining what you have worked for is just as worthy and valuable as moving forwards** in your goal achievement.

Flexibility with Macros and Micros

Flexibility with Macros means to be more laid-back in your approach to your daily carbohydrate/fats/protein and fibre intakes. Being flexible with your micronutrients means the same thing in terms of vitamins and minerals. You don't have to be perfect every day, but if you are good 80-90% of the time it is probably the best way. Even being better 50% of the time will have greater effect than not doing anything at all. It is about consistency, which comes from the ability to maintain something, which comes from it being psychologically sound and flexible - which this diet is. Let us have a look further into flexibility regarding macronutrients.

Caloric Flexibility

If we were to think more in terms of weekly allowances of calories, we could be much more flexible with how we distribute them. For example, if you ate more calories one day, you could easily re-distribute (shuffle) some calories around during the week to allow for/compensate for it, should you desire. As we have already discussed, this is not always necessary; you could always simply call it a 'maintenance day' and then continue as normal next day.

But feel free to move the calories around as you see fit – if you wish to eat more one day and less the next, keep daily calorie intake more consistent daily, shift calories around in your day so you eat more at preferred time etc. The main goal is to make the diet yours, and to design it in a way which makes you adhere to it as much as possible.

With that said, we should caution against extremes. Although we have relatively large flexibility in how we distribute our weekly calories, I would recommend staying in a low calorie pattern for no longer than 2 days at a time. For example, I wouldn't like to see someone eat 500 calories a day throughout the week, and then have a massive caloric splurge on the weekend – such a prolonged caloric deficit may have problems for metabolism, and you may struggle to maintain nutrient quality throughout the week.

Protein Flexibility

For the most part, we are trying to aim for a certain amount of protein per day. We also want to get a share of fats and carbohydrates without cutting anything out. Regarding protein, this is probably the least flexible of options. You should try, where you can, to maintain at least the recommended 0.8 grams of protein per pound of bodyweight. This macronutrient should be kept in the desired range in as many days as possible on a more consistent basis.

I would also try to keep your protein intake relatively stable on low and high days. It would be more preferable to change the amounts of carbohydrates and fats on low days, rather than change the protein. Protein seems to be more important when the body is in a dieting state, so cutting protein on a low calorie day could prove more detrimental.

However, we need to be realistic and flexible with this. You are not going to be able to hit your protein target every single day. For example, if you are to do a full day or partial fast, you will likely get nowhere near it. Don't fret – one day without sufficient protein is not going to make all of your lean body mass fall off. In fact, many of the alternate day dieting studies showed better lean mass retention.

I would certainly recommend, where possible, to get as close to your desired protein amount on partial fasting days, as it will also help with satiety during those times (protein is better for satiety). But please understand, if you have a day without desired protein intake (even when not fasting), it is not going to completely ruin everything. It's only when we consistently skip or neglect protein intake that we will create less than optimal results.

Carbohydrate/Fats Flexibility

Regarding carbohydrates, there is a lot more flexibility to be had. You can abstain fully from carbohydrates one day if you wish. This could allow you to have that 'quota' on a different day. For example, a person who cuts out 400 calories of carbohydrates on a low day, could move them to a high calorie day – meaning a massive carbohydrate meal. This can actually be quite effective, especially when timed around/after workouts when carbohydrate consumption is more beneficial. Obviously you would still try to maintain your daily calorie allowance in doing so. The type of carbohydrates you eat are also your choice; fast or slow digesting is no problem, as we have seen.

Even though we are allowing freedom of choice with carbohydrates, do not take too many liberties. We still have micronutrient quotas to meet, and 'quality' carbohydrates from whole wheat (unless you have an allergy) and vegetable/fruit sources are the best ways to hit these. But even with micronutrients, one day of poor eating every now and again is not going to hinder your success, as long as the rest of the time you are hitting/exceeding your recommended intakes. This goes the same for fibre. Ideally we would maintain consistent levels of fibre, but you are not going to die if you fall short one day.

Regarding fats – it is no surprise that we also should maintain flexibility here. I would avoid cutting out fats from your diet altogether, as they are needed for hormonal health and vitamin absorption. However, should you desire to have a more carbohydrate heavy day one day, feel free to shift the carb/fat ratio around as desired.

Section 3 - Mental

Introduction to Mental

Let's face it. We can all lose weight if we want to. If someone offered you a million dollars to lose 10 pounds, I have no doubt that almost everyone would have this weight lost in a month, maximum. Why is that? We must understand that weight loss is mostly mental; if we have the motivation to do, it we don't even need to know how to do it perfectly; almost everyone knows instinctively how to lose weight. It's often purely a matter of motivation - wanting it enough.

We have looked so far about the 'how' of dieting. We have shattered myths that would otherwise halt your success. Now is the time to work on the mental side of the diet. This doesn't mean lying down on a couch while telling a psychologist all your food nightmares. It is simply working out exactly what you want, why you want it, what is standing in your way, creating a plan and then assessing that plan. We need to create motivation before you can do anything; a drive that will see you achieve your goal. While most diet books lack this vital component, you are about to embark on discovering the real reason for a diet being successful.

Although I considered putting this part of the book at the very beginning, it is placed here for a reason. The planning part of this section requires that you understand the diet fully, and I want you to leave this book with an unstoppably high level of motivation and belief that you can achieve you weight loss dreams. At the end of this section of the book, you will be so enthused that nothing will stand in your way. What you are about to read is very powerful information - it can be applied not only to your dieting goals, but to all aspects of your life.

Chapter 11
Goal Setting

Goal setting works. It has been proven time and time again that the people with the clearest goals achieve more than those without goals, or those that have less apparent goals. Sure, some people get lucky and fall into success without trying hard or without knowing where they are going in life (we all know one or two of those people). But those are the exceptions to the rule, not the rule. If we sit on our behinds all day complaining that other people are 'lucky', that it always goes right for them, or that they were just born into opportunity, we will do ourselves a great disservice. Please remember that you only live once - just one life to make things how you want them to be. You have the biggest influence over your life than any other thing, especially in modern society. Let's aim for our best life ever, and be the best version of ourselves.

Goal setting works on a multitude of levels. It directs your awareness to information that will help you in your quest, and away from things that will be detrimental to you succeeding. When you hear a new word or phrase for the first time, it is often heightened in our subconscious. For the next few days or weeks it seems as though everywhere you go the new phrase is following you. You hear it on the news, read it in the paper, see it on web pages etc. But it is not that the new information is now surrounding you; it has always been there. However, now your subconscious has become more aware of the phrase, it will filter out more information pertaining to it and place it right there in your conscious mind. Goal setting works much in the same way. By consciously creating a goal, you are setting up a situation where your subconscious mind will filter out information, leaving you with a higher chance of succeeding in your quest. Goal setting also serves as a highly motivating and energizing force.

Excite Yourself

The goals you set should be ones that excite you. As long as you believe they are possible to achieve, a high goal is very motivating, and often provides more success than smaller, more achievable goals. Aim for the stars, and you will at least reach the moon! Goal setting also increases your perseverance in trying to achieve what you want. People who set goals in the right manner are much more likely to see them through to the end. This works by increasing our commitment to our goal and our dreams; often the biggest key to success is sheer determination and tenacity. By evaluating our goals regularly, we are putting ourselves in a situation that amplifies our willpower and self control.

I am not a happy-clappy positive thinker, I am a realist. I don't think that you can be the fastest person in the world, make a multi-billion-dollar empire or become the next Albert Einstein. But I do believe that everyone can become their natural healthy weight and achieve a lot of success in their lives, and so you should believe this too. Almost every successful person follows a certain path; whether they do this consciously, or whether it is more of an innate process doesn't matter. It can be learned and copied so that you can achieve a much higher rate of success.

Most people reading this think they know what they want. To a certain extent they do, they are just not **clear** enough on it. Goals need to be very specific; a goal that is too general is not an effective one. People state things such as "I want to lose weight" or "I don't want to be as fat any more". Unfortunately, these people never seem to reach their goal. Occasionally you come across someone who gets closer to the mark and states something such as "I'm going to get my body in shape for beach season", and while this is a more specific goal, it is still far from perfect. Below is how your goal should ideally be stated

"I have lost 15 pounds over the last 10 weeks and my body is now in the best shape it has been for years, just in time for my holiday"

What is so special about the above quote? How does it trump the other statements? Well, for a start, it is stated in the positive. It is very important that you highlight exactly what you *do* want rather than what you don't. The subconscious cannot use the negative form as efficiently. An example of this would be a person who says "I don't want to mess up my presentation". This person who repeats this mantra will end up causing stress and anxiety as their subconscious is visualizing messing up. They would then have a greater likelihood to produce the undesired effect of messing up the presentation - an effect known as a 'self-fulfilling prophecy'. It would be much more effective to say "I want to give the best presentation I have ever given". As this is stated positively, the subconscious now brings up images of delivering a stunning performance, thus leading to less nerves and anxiety, thus promoting the likelihood of making a great presentation. This effect is often understood by sportspeople, such as a tennis player who says "don't hit it in the net" before a serve. If they don't fulfil their prophecy, you can be assured that they will still find a different way to mess up the shot.

The previous quote is also stated as if it has already been achieved. This has a subtle, yet powerful effect on how our subconscious processes the goal. Take a look at the following statement.

"I would like to lose 15 pounds over the next 10 weeks so my body is in shape for my holiday".

Although it is technically the same goal, as it is said in future terms it has a much smaller effect on your arousal. It is weak and almost emotionless. The only emotion it seems to stir is that the goal is 10 weeks away, rather than already completed. Compare the two phrases again for yourself and see. It seems as if the quote in the present 'already achieved' sense fires you up more.

It also has the added benefit of helping alter your subconscious beliefs - a vital component to you changing. Lots of times we self-sabotage as our subconscious beliefs do not match our conscious goals. For example, if I were to say that I want to become a top athlete, but I don't fully believe I can do it, then this will create a conscious/subconscious conflict to which I will be more likely to self-sabotage. By stating it as if it is already achieved, "I am a top athlete", it has a more profound effect on our belief system (over time) and hence our ability to achieve it improves. This works in a number of ways, but the main manner for its functionality is that we start to consciously and subconsciously visualize the task as already achieved. The more we do that, the more we send the message to our brain that it is possible as we have already done it (we haven't, but we are trying to fool our brain into thinking that we have).

The above goal is also very specific. It states numbers, and it is also time-based or has some sort of deadline attached to it. This is important as it gives a heightened sense of urgency. As a rule, set the deadline **before** you actually want to achieve it. For example, if your holiday is in 12 weeks, set the deadline for 10 weeks, as it allows 2 weeks of flexibility should something go wrong (such as an illness) which could potentially slow down your progress. Flexibility with your goals is important, as an inflexible system will produce more stress and more chance of a complete derailment should something crop up unexpectedly. The specific numbers that you set for weight loss (or inches lost around your waist, for example) enables us to measure, record and evaluate it more effectively. Your evaluation will become a vital constituent of your success, as we will see later on. So make sure that your goal has something that you can measure.

Dream Big, but Not Too Big

Every goal must also have a certain level of push to it. It should drive you and be big enough to excite you, but be wary. A goal that is too great can be more demoralizing and un-motivational. This is a tricky balance to meet, but there are a few rules you should follow to ensure the goal set is right for you.

Make sure that your goal is first and foremost realistic. For example, losing 10 pounds in a week is highly unrealistic (although, in rare circumstances, possible). If you were to set this goal, you would probably be sorely disappointed with your results and end up giving up. Losing a total of 5 pounds in 12 weeks, on the other hand (although very realistic and achievable), does not excite enough. This could potentially fail on the grounds of not being challenging enough. When a task is deemed as too easy by the person, often it is not achieved as we lose awareness.

Think about performing a sport or game against someone who is well below our skill level. We will often make many more mistakes than normal against them, as we deem the task of beating them too easy; although we may still win, our performance suffers dramatically. If the goal you have set sparks some arousal when you read it, then it is probably demanding enough. Losing between 1 or 2 pounds per week is realistic, achievable by most, without being too demanding, and over a long period of time can amount to huge weight losses. If you were to aim for 2 pounds per week of weight loss, even if you only hit half that amount you would be 50 pounds lighter in a year. Aim high, push your boundaries, but please stay on planet earth in the process.

There is also a motivational statement within the goal. We all need a **'why'** or our goal is doomed to fail. If there is a 'why' (and it is arousing enough), then we can use *that* as our focus in times of low motivation. The previous goal uses an upcoming holiday as the motivational force. Whenever enthusiasm is low, we can focus on our holiday and use the visuals of our holiday to prevent any situations that would sabotage our success. For example, if you want to raid the cookie jar and blow your diet, spending a couple of minutes (or even seconds) thinking about your holiday will quickly quell any cravings. If the 'why' is inspiring enough, you won't even need the visualization for it to work, it will be there subconsciously.

Long Term/Short Term

Within your goals you should also think long term. This helps us to dream big while staying within the realms of possibility. You should also break these long term goals down by setting medium and short term goals, starting with the biggest goal first and working your way back.

I once heard a story about a mountain climber suffering a fall and breaking his leg. Stuck in the wilderness and miles away from the nearest village with no contact seemed like a dead end, literally. But this wounded man dragged himself along the ground for miles until he reached the nearest village and was taken to hospital, where he recovered fully. Astounded by his story, when questioned about how he managed to do this amazing feat of endurance, he answered very interestingly. The goal, or the big picture, was to get to the village which was miles away. Although we couldn't call this an exciting goal as such, it was definitely a necessity, and motivation to achieve this goal was high. But the interesting thing was that he broke it down into smaller manageable goals. "If I can just get to that tree 100 meters away" was followed by "If I can just get to that rock 100 meters away" and so forth. This was broken down further into a mini game. By guessing how many 'drags' it would take to get to the nearest checkpoint and then counting, he created a process that focussed his mind on the task in hand *now*.

This is a perfect analogy for how goal setting should work. See the big picture, the ultimate goal which will essentially inspire you and motivate you throughout. Any time you lose enthusiasm, focus on that end goal and what it means to you. But by breaking it down into smaller more manageable chunks you make the task seem much more achievable. It fills the gap between the 'here' and the 'there'. By working out what you have to do to achieve these smaller checkpoints/goals, we become what we call 'process oriented'. Our mind is focussed on the task in hand to achieve the goal. Enough talk, let us look at an example.

Example

We have an example of a 35 year old man who is 100 pounds overweight, severely obese. His health is suffering, and he knows he simply cannot stay this way forever and decides to make a change. Here is what his goal setting should look like.

"I am 40 years old and I have lost 100 pounds since my heaviest. I am much happier, healthier and enjoy life much more as a result. I feel like a new man, my wife and kids look up to me as a role model, which fills me with a sense of great satisfaction and pride".

This is the long term goal, the big picture. This is aiming for the stars. Losing 100 pounds is a huge deal and anyone setting this goal knows it. This goal will be the ultimate driving force behind all of your actions, ultimately leading to your success. Is it a challenging goal – definitely. Losing 100 pounds is never an easy task. Is it achievable – very. 100 pounds over 5 years works out as less than half a pound per week. While weight loss does not occur as predictably as we would like, over such a long time period we have enough time to make adjustments and create a lot of flexibility. While plateaus often occur in weight loss, as long as (in general) we keep ahead of the schedule, it gives us a buffer to work with. Now we should look at breaking it down further.

"I have lost 40 pounds this year. My clothes fit better than ever and everyone is commenting on how good I look. Some people don't even recognize me when they see me"

Again, this is a great goal for several reasons. Stated in the positive as if it has already been achieved, it also includes many highly motivational factors. It can clearly be converted into an image of walking around, meeting people and feeling great about yourself. While it is a big goal, over a year it still works out as less than 1 pound a week. We should still aim to keep ahead of this schedule as it will give us that buffer. But if we don't, then we can still be on track for our ultimate goal. Even half of this weight loss is what is necessary to achieve the ultimate goal of 100 pounds over 5 years. This would be considered a long – medium term goal. Now let us get a smaller picture.

"I have reached my 12-week goal weight by losing 15 pounds by (insert date here). I have gone down a pant size, and I

am already feeling lighter on my toes. My back pain has started to go and I feel 10 years younger in my fitness levels. I am so much happier; this is really exciting"

We have broken it down into a manageable chunk; this is the equivalent of creating those checkpoints. This is our 'tree' or 'rock' that we are scrambling towards. It is different to the other goals because it is more in sight - a goal that is well in reach. 12 weeks is a time period that is very easy to visualize happening, and as a result is very motivating, not for its magnitude, but for the fact it is very evident. By setting a 12 week goal of losing 15 pounds (just over a pound a week) we could potentially lose 60 pound in a year. At this rate we would lose our ultimate dream goal of 100 pounds in less than 2 years. But this is not the way to think about it, we need to create checkpoints, buffers and places we can get to so we can rest for a moment. Our injured climber didn't just go from one checkpoint to the next continuously. After reaching the checkpoint, a small rest and evaluation was necessary before continuing, and this is the same for our goals. When you reach certain checkpoints, you will need to stabilize yourself mentally and physically, maintaining that position for a small while before setting off on your next achievement. This will be covered more fully in our chapter on 'periodization'.

Maybe your goal is not to lose 100 pounds. Maybe it is to lose more, or maybe just 10 pounds is all you are after. But in any case, you should always look to set at least one dream goal - the ultimate idea of where you want to be. As long as you believe it is possible, dream as big as you can. From there, break it down into smaller, manageable chunks.

Chapter Summary

Set your sights high. Create a goal that inspires you utterly; a really big goal. However, set it far enough in the future that it is completely achievable. For example, losing 100 pounds is a great goal, but if you say to do it in one year you may end up giving up as it seems too difficult. Doing it over 5 years is not so far out in the future that it seems a distant wish, but not too short a time period that it seems impossible.

Break this big goal into smaller, more manageable chunks. Look for an ultimate goal, a 1-year goal, and a 3 (12 week) month goal.

State your goals as if you have already achieved them. "I am 10 pounds thinner than 2 months ago" is better than saying "I would like to lose 10 pounds in 2 months". It takes a big step in changing our subconscious beliefs.

State your goals in positive and specific terms. "I don't want to be overweight anymore" is not a positive or a specific goal. Use dates and times to set yourself deadlines, and use numbers of exactly how much you wish to lose (or what you wish to weigh).

Allow your goals to have buffers within them, this allows for flexibility should something go wrong. For example, if you wish to lose 50 pounds in 2 years, your 1-year goal should be to lose 35 pounds, and your 12-week goal should be to lose 12 pounds. You aim to lose a little more than you wish to in order to achieve your ultimate goal.

Chapter 12
Motivation

Creating a set of goals that are inspiring goes a long way towards motivating you. As you went through the goal setting process, especially in setting your ultimate goal, you undoubtedly felt as if you are ready to start there and then. Well go for it; you should set in motion your success as soon as possible, with whatever small action possible at the time.

But motivation often dwindles after time. One of the problems with getting closer to our goals is that our drive slows down as we realize we are succeeding. There are many reasons for this, some of which we will address. But this section is all about keeping that fire going, maintaining the will to succeed. Whether you are failing in your attempt to achieve what you set out to do, or whether you are over-achieving, keeping our motivation high enables us to get where we want. We will look at how you can use some simple tricks that amplify your desires and keep you going through the tougher times.

The diet itself makes the whole process much easier. Having to only effectively diet for one day, followed by a feeding day, means that you only really have to keep your motivation high on those low days. Say, for example, on your low calories day you start to feel a few hunger pangs and get the urge to splurge, just remembering that tomorrow you are allowed to eat much more than normal will enable you to continue. You only have to grind it out for a day, or even until your next meal really. Also, as we are not eliminating any foods from our diet, it makes it a lot easier to stick to. We can use the foods we love to eat as rewards for doing well the previous day, which is highly motivating. By utilizing intermittent fasting or meal skipping, we are still allowed bigger meals at other points in the day, effectively making each day only a half day diet. Later on, we will also discuss how to set up your long term goals so that you get well earned breaks from the diet, where you are not going backwards but just staying at the same level for a short time to stabilize and re-charge your motivation. The more we can see this as a longer term plan, the bigger the goals we can achieve with less effort.

The Why

We all deep down know what we want, but it is simply not enough; you need to also figure out *why* you want it. We all know those people who would like to lose weight and always talk about it but never achieve it. Maybe you are one of those people, always saying that you wish you could lose those few pounds. You will never achieve anything with this type of mind-set. For a start your goal is not exciting enough, and not specific enough, so go back to the last section and read it clearly and set some better goals. But the real reason for your failures and inability to change are subconscious. Often our subconscious feels too comfortable at a certain place. The longer we spend there, the more comfortable we get and the harder it is to make a change. There is also an inner push/pull happening; You are being pushed away from your goal and pulled towards it all the time. Depending on which focus is greater at the time determines whether you succeed or not in the long term. We need to tip the balance in favour of succeeding more often.

Some factors push us towards our goal, like our doctor telling us to lose weight or our health will suffer. Sometimes someone could make a negative comment that pushes us towards our goal, sometimes we can just have the drive to get ourselves into that old dress. We need to identify these factors in order to change our focus when we start losing motivation. You are most probably focussing on the wrong things when your success starts slipping. If we can also identify the things that will block our success, then we can also take actions to prevent or limit their influence. Just remember

"you will not achieve your goal if you don't know why you want it, or if your reason is not inspiring enough"

Take 5 minutes out, with a pencil and paper. This will be the most life changing 5 minutes of your life, so stop reading now and go collect your note writing equipment. Have them yet? Ok, write down as many reasons as you can for losing weight. What are you going to get out of it? Here are some examples

Feel confident
More attractive
Fit into that old dress
I have increased risk of Cancer
Less joint pain
Be a role model for my kids
I have an increased risk of CAD
Re-gain control of my life
Be happier
Look good in wedding photos
Improve fertility
Achieve a goal
I am at increased risk of diabetes
Lower chance of injury
Live longer
Help sporting performance
Make family proud
Better health

Do you have enough reasons yet? Look at your list, find the ones which are more emotional for you. Perhaps it is a positive emotion – such as imagining being more confident. Perhaps it is a negative emotion, such as joint pain – you can use both positive and negative emotions to motivate you. Keep asking yourself "why" for each reason. Why does that mean so much to you? What will it give you? Why is it so important to you? Keep asking "why" until you cannot go any further. As an example, choosing 'improve fertility,

"I really want kids one day, and losing the weight will improve my chances of having my dream family."

This is an example of positive motivation; you are using a positive example to direct you towards your goals. This in itself can be a very powerful form of motivation. We have also come to a deeper realization of why we want to lose weight; the real reasons are bigger than just seeing numbers fly off the scale. To affect areas of your life such as health and children is a real wake up call. Let us look at another example, 'live longer'.

"By improving my health and losing weight I am improving my chances of living longer. I want to live longer so that I can see my children develop into full adults, and even see them have children. I would love to be a big part of the lives of my grandchildren, looking after them would provide great pleasure. I would love to impart my life wisdom upon them and be to them what my grandparents were to me. I also want to live a full life with my beloved wife, experience as much as I can of the world with her. But most of all, I want to make sure she is safe and secure as I am there to look after her."

This is, again, a goal that goes much deeper than just saying "live longer". If you have children, thinking about their futures and looking after them longer, and even seeing your grandchildren and playing an important role in their life may be a hugely motivational force for you. Maybe the last line, talking about looking after your loved one, hits home a little stronger. Losing weight is not the only goal – there are a multitude of deeper benefits. So for every reason that you have for losing weight, keep asking why. More and more reasons should extend from that single statement. When you have hit the reason that strikes the biggest chord with you, you have found an emotional connection with your goal; this is important as it will be our main focus during the process.

Take that sheet of paper with your reasons, attach it to your sheet of goals, now pin those sheets to your fridge door, bathroom mirror or, better still, put a digital copy on your computer desktop image. This way it will be in your face constantly, seeping into your conscious and subconscious. Nothing builds motivation and success like constantly being reminded of what you want and why you want it.

Using Negatives

It is quite simple, if you are completely happy or satisfied with where you are now, you will not have the motivation to change. We have evolved to try and use the least amount of physical and mental energy possible. Wherever we can, we try to avoid anything that would cause us strain and make us have to actually work something. Add to that the quick fix societal memes that are spreading worldwide, and we are getting into a right mess. What really causes people to get fired up and actually do something? Why do we procrastinate so much as a species?

Procrastination is actually a very useful tool. It enables us to use negative motivation, a state where we are motivated to work purely from the fact we want to avoid negative consequences. For example, if you know you need to do a presentation for work but seem to be whittling away the time, your motivation will peak right about the time you have no time left. In the end, you get it done in record time, and just wonder why you didn't get started on it earlier and get it out of the way. When there is too much time, or it's not a bad enough situation, our brain tells us to conserve as much energy as possible; worst thing would be to get the presentation completed and out of the way only to find out we don't need to do it anymore. By procrastinating, we build up our motivation until it is at tipping point, and then we can do anything. We can also use this negative motivation to our benefit.

The problem with positive motivation is that it is much weaker for some people. It really depends where you are at a certain time regarding your progress, and also personality has a lot to do with it. To most people, although setting a goal is very inspiring, usually greater success comes from the depths of despair. We can get great motivation in looking to how we 'want to live'; imagining all the things we can do, have and be can be very pleasing and leave us with a sense of "I really should do that". But there is a big difference between "I should" and "I must". "I must" comes from a need, not a desire - a fiery Will that cannot be contained. Only you can decide what motivates you more at this point in time. Does working towards an 'ideal' create a sense of urgency in you, or is it more likely to manifest itself from a necessity to get away from something negative? The person who says "I'll show them" is capable of big things - just make sure you channel it in a positive way.

But on the whole, people seem to do greater things when faced with negative motivation. For example, most people will be more likely to make a change in their weight when they get to the point where "this is simply not good enough anymore". They see a horrible photo of themselves next to other people, or an embarrassing situation where they can't fit into a plane seat, or someone unfortunately says something cruel and unkind. Maybe their old wedding dress is 2,3 or more sizes too small for them now, and they despise what they have become. While I personally hate to see these situations happen for people, and feel great sympathy for them, it is actually serving a greater purpose. If it means that someone feels really bad about themselves for a week, but they gain a lifetime of pleasure from the success of getting where they want to, then those negative situations are all for the good. But there are two types of personalities. One who takes this negative and turns it into fuel to fire up their motivation, and the other that becomes a victim of their own failures. Which one are you? Do you blame everyone else and everything else other than yourself for your failures? Or do you take control of the things that you can control and make something of yourself. Usually the people who don't accept responsibility are the ones who don't feel it is possible for them to achieve what they want. By reading through this book, you have a way that you definitely can achieve success.

In every negative there is a lesson. We should take that lesson, learn from it, move on, and hopefully we don't make the same mistake again. If you do this, you can be successful in every aspect of life. On the other hand, if you dwell on your failures and become a victim, blaming everything else around you, then you will be doomed to fail over and over again. Perspective is the key here; successful people see failures in a completely different light. I don't have to tell you about how the invention of the light bulb came after over 1000 failures, or the hundreds of entrepreneurs who came from rock bottom to build multi-million dollar empires. It seems that almost every example of successful weight loss I see comes with a negative driving force. The fat kid who was bullied at school and has since lost all the weight, or the girl who lost her boyfriend and then went on to lose pounds too. Or the guy who used to be athletic, ate themselves into depression and obesity, and then with a dramatic turning point in their lives (usually seeing themselves in a photo compared to how they used to be) gets their lean body back again and has a newfound philosophy on life. Shakira's voice coach told her she sounded like a dying goat and would not make anything of herself, J.K. Rowling was rejected several times before finding a publisher for the now famous 'Harry Potter' series.

This is a quote from Lynn Haraldson, author of Lynnsweigh blog and someone who lost 170 pounds of weight. This was the tipping point, the thing that woke her up, forcing her to realize that this simply was not good enough.

"I didn't like how I was feeling. I'd been thin before. I missed that. I missed being active. Also, I didn't like how I looked. I went, 'I think it's time.' I had to really look at the photographs. I looked at the pictures and finally it got painful enough that I knew I needed to really, really do something"

Notice how the motivation was painful. This is an example of how someone used a negative emotion as fire to go on and achieve her dream. Here is another great example of using a negative experience to your advantage. Cammy, the owner of Tippytoediet.com and loser of 100 pounds in weight had this to say.

"A friend of mine had to have triple bypass surgery. Shortly after that, I went to my doctor for bronchitis and he paused when he had the stethoscope over my heart and said, 'I would like you to go do a treadmill test.' The doctor said I might need angioplasty. I got so worked up and they couldn't fit me in for three weeks. I was encouraged because obviously I wasn't facing imminent death, but I thought, this is just what happened to my friend. *I was just frantic and I worked myself up so that my blood pressure was out of control. I had to go to the doctor to get a tranquilizer kind of thing just to calm myself down. And I thought,* I do not

want to ever go through this again *as far as knowing that the way I was living my life was likely contributing to something like that, that all these choices were catching up to me.*

"It turned out someone misread the test results... I think the kicker was I did all that worrying, all of that imagining the most dire thing, and the whole time telling myself, **you could have done something about this years ago.** *It was a great lesson. I would never want to go through it again. But if I faced it again now I would be able to say, 'No, I eat right, I get plenty of exercise. There may be a problem here but it's not because I haven't been trying to take care of myself.' I took control back there and I think that was the issue before is I didn't have control of my life."*

Again, a negative, even frightening experience was used to supercharge the motivation of a person. Using this reason, Cammy managed to lose the weight in just 17 months. What is your reason, your 'why' and your motivation? Think hard about it, because it will likely be the difference between your success and failure.

Often, and in the case of Lynn, people finally 'see' themselves. What does this mean? The human mind is very adept at blocking out any information that would be painful to them. Many people unconsciously choose not to see themselves as they are. One of my good friends recently lost a lot of weight, and when we were talking about his motivation he told me that he had seen a photo of himself next to his friends. He finally saw the proportions of himself against others, and was shocked. "But you see yourself every day in the mirror" I said. He replied "Yes, but your mind can easily play tricks on you. I knew I was big, but my mind seemed to ignore it, especially as there was no one else to compare against".

Bodybuilders can often suffer from this, seeing themselves as smaller and less muscular than they actually are, or the reverse is seen in Anorexia, where painfully thin people see themselves as much bigger than they are. We all experience it to some extent. One day we look in the mirror and see ourselves as satisfactory (or some people see themselves as amazing). Other days, sometimes even hours later, we can look in the mirror and see our worst nightmare. It is highly unlikely that our body is changing that quickly, but our perceptions can change in a moment. Stand around in a waiting room at an obesity clinic and you are likely to walk away feeling rather good about yourself. However, spend time reading a magazine filled with glamorous models and 'bikini babes' and the same body you possess is likely to be perceived very differently. Just like the illusion of a Necker cube, our mind can flip our perception of our own bodies. It is all about what we compare against, but if there is nothing to compare with, how can we tell if our minds are not playing tricks on us? This is where we can be a little clever and use this 'trick of the mind' to our own advantage.

Vision Board

Before we do this, it is important to note that although we have seen that negative motivation can be a very powerful tool to drive us towards our goal, the downside is that it can be confidence knocking. There is a way of using both sides of the coin to our advantage however; by cycling between the negative, confidence knocking but highly motivating state, and the confidence/happiness building state, we can achieve the drive we want without the bad effects. Most people do this naturally to some extent, but we are taking control of the mechanisms here for our own benefit. The strategy presented to you here can be used for anything in life.

What we are going to do is collect a few photographs. You can do this digitally by scouring the internet, or manually by making a scrapbook. First, get a photo of yourself that you simply hate. This will probably be more difficult than you would imagine, as you have most likely thrown them all out. Nevertheless, find the worst one you can and place it in the centre of your scrapbook page, or create a file on your computer and copy and paste it in. If you simply can't find one that is emotional enough, then make one in the most unflattering pose you can. Next, place images of fit, healthy bodies around it; make sure that the images are deemed achievable by yourself. The images should be something you believe is possible for you, given a long time and a lot of motivation, but not so high that you think it is a pipe dream. Even use an old picture of yourself.

This is your motivation page/board. Some people call this a 'vision board', and they can be highly motivating. This vision board is also going to fill you with some negative emotion too; this is natural. Prepare to be disappointed with yourself, and prepare for some guilty feelings to start to emerge. This is your subconscious building up a level of motivation that will be unstoppable. It is some very powerful stuff, and I make no apologies for the negative emotions you will experience. There is a higher purpose to all of this; this is about more than just your current fleeting feelings, this is your health and life we are talking about. Feeling good emotionally has taken you into your current physical state. Whether it was emotional eating, or lack of awareness as to what was happening to your body, the immediate pleasure of food has made you ignore the reality. It is time to reverse it. This vision board is going to be your main tool for powering your motivation. You will need to place this somewhere you can see it every day, like the door of the fridge. Dedicate at least one minute a day, or several times a day, to just standing in front of it and looking at it. Why not combine it with your goal sheet, reading through your goals shortly afterwards. This small time investment will have an incredible impact on your life.

The Success Board

Using our vision board can be very powerful. However, if we stay in this state forever, it can be damaging. In the short term, a few weeks of doing this will not hurt you, but if it develops into a full blown habit then it can lead to a life of discontent. Often, some of the greatest achievers in life can still be left unhappy. This ability to get down on yourself and use these negative emotions can be very powerful in achievement, but the effect it has on your confidence and happiness can also take its toll. This is where we are going to balance it with another vision board, or rather a 'success board'. At first, this will have no value. But with time, and with every successive achievement, this will be more and more powerful and lead to greater happiness and contentment with your life. Here is how it works.

When you have achieved your first checkpoint goal – perhaps 12 weeks into your diet for example – make a new photo of yourself. You can put yourself in the same pose as before, but try to be more flattering. Even sucking the gut in a little, or standing in a way that is more aesthetically pleasing. Use better lighting, nicer fitting clothing and anything else you can think of to make yourself look better. Place this photo next to your 'bad photo' in a 'before and after' style. If the difference is not visible enough (sometimes even 15 pounds of weight loss is not noticeable in a photo), place other images of people with even worse bodies around it. By comparing yourself to images that are worse than your body, you are building up your confidence. When your new photo gets to a stage where there is a noticeable difference between the before and after, it will start to create a form of positive motivation, as well as a confidence boost.

You could also put images of foods that you wish to eat more of, such as vegetables, on the outskirts of this success board, or images of people exercising. This board will start to create a deep rooted connection between the 'new you' and a feeling of success and happiness, as well as the good habits which got you there. But it will do it in a way that doesn't hamper your success - it builds upon it. The better your 'new you' photo becomes, the more you will be filled with a sense of motivational satisfaction.

Use this success board sparingly at first. For one, it will have little impact until the 'after' image is significantly better than the 'before' image. But over time you will see that it has a profound effect on your mood and positive motivation. For some people, it puts them into a mood that is 'too contented' with themselves. If you feel your goal achievement is reaching a plateau (and your adherence or motivation to stick to the diet has been the reason), then use this board less, choosing to focus on your vision board more. At first, use the vision board much more often, almost exclusively. Then when you start to achieve your goals you can begin to integrate the success board sparingly. When you are at your desired goal (if you are completely happy), you could use each board 50% of the time. Even create a single board that shows only your before and after picture with nothing else. The negative picture will be viewed as a 'you' that you don't ever wish to become again. The new picture will be compared against the old in a way that makes you grateful of how much you have achieved and how far you have come. This is a happy balance that will keep you motivated to maintain what you have strived to achieve, yet not at the expense of your confidence. A person who has dieted down to 160 pounds is far happier with their lives than a person who has let themselves go from 130 pounds to 160 pounds. The difference is perception and what their focus is.

Social Accountability

This is yet another way of using that push/pull or positive and negative motivation to help us in our success. Social accountability is basically bringing friends and family or work colleagues in on the plan. With today's social networking online, you can even set up social accountability with people you don't know.

In order to use this principle, you are going to have to find ways of letting people know exactly what you are doing, let them know that you are going on a diet and why. This works in two ways. Hopefully, for the most part, the people around you are going to support you through it, helping you out where they can. This helps keep your motivation on track, as no one likes to show they are incapable of doing something they set out to do. If you fall of the bandwagon with your diet, it is all too easy to keep it to yourself and completely lose motivation. This is often the reason we don't tell people what we are planning to do. We are so afraid of failing in front of everyone that we keep our goals to ourselves, but the problem is that it becomes a self-fulfilling prophecy. But if everyone else knows about it, it gives you the internal drive to jump back on the weight-loss train again and try your best.

Unfortunately, sometimes the support is not there, and there may even be people who create a negative environment. We all know the people at the office who sneer anytime someone says they are going to do something that they clearly can't achieve. These are the same people that say nothing when that person has achieved their goal. Why do people do this? There is an innate drive in humans to try and keep everyone on an even keel. Someone who is perceived as an equal should not be able to accomplish something that another can't do. So often, people try to knock others down, sabotage their efforts or find another way to make themselves feel better. But there is balance in the universe, and just like the vision board can be used to direct negative emotions positively, we can use these people in our lives to ignite our drive. Why not add a picture of their face to your vision board? "I'll show them".

There are some common forms of social accountability that you can take advantage of, some work much better than others; people can achieve great things when a lot of people are counting on them. The most basic form is to tell everyone and anyone that you are going on a diet. While some people naturally do this, others are a little more reluctant. If this is you, get out of your shell and tell as many people as you can; if it makes the difference between success and failure it is worthwhile. The only fear you have is that you won't succeed. But the only reason you wouldn't succeed is lack of motivation, and this gives you a boost in exactly that.

You could also set up a blog or website/page which documents your dieting. Many people follow others dieting in the hopes that they can find something that will work for them. By seeing others being successful, it is a good test to see if the diet works before they put in energy. I call this 'theoretical dieting' and many people partake in this. Soon, after setting up your page, you could have many followers offering advice, words of encouragement and making you accountable to them as motivation. You could also do this type of activity in an online forum, to which there are many dealing with weight loss. Don't forget to promote this diet (wink).

What about taking it a step further and setting up a training/diet partner? Using each other for encouragement and motivation can be a great spark to your success. Pick someone who is equally motivated; if you don't know anyone then tell them to read this section of the book and they will be fired up in no time. By working out with a partner, or just having someone to check in with periodically (ideally every 2 days or once a week at the least), you can have someone to push you when you are down, and someone to share your highs when you are up. There is also an element of guilt when your partner is doing so well and you are not. There is nothing like a little guilt to whip your behind back into shape (literally). And if you are motivated by competition, why not set up a challenge between yourselves. See who can stay the course the longest, even having some money on it can double the effectiveness of this strategy.

Another way to take the competition idea to the next level is to enter a body transformation challenge. There are lots of these created and undertaken every year. Supplement companies do them as a means to promote a new product, and some fitness blogs and websites do them purely to promote themselves. They can be a great way to have a clear defined goal in mind, something definite that you can commit to. Another variant of this is to do it for charity. By losing weight for a cause that is bigger than your own (and for something that you feel is worthwhile), you can create a clear and motivating 'why' that inspires and drives you. Getting people to follow your success online can encourage you to stay the course fully, and as it is for a good cause, you are more likely to get positive re-enforcement from others.

The Morning Ritual

We now have a few tactics for improving our motivation. Setting up our lives so that we are more accountable to achieve our goal obviously works, but make yourself accountable to yourself. You have a responsibility to keep yourself in as good health as possible. No one else is going to do it for you, it is all in your power and largely controlled by your motivation and focus.

The best way to ensure that you are adding logs to the fire every day is to commit to one small act that helps you on your path. The act of looking at your vision board every single morning takes only one minute, sometimes less. But if you do it religiously, you will definitely experience the positive effects of it. Include all aspects of motivation every morning and you are not only throwing logs on the fire, but dousing those logs in gasoline.

Start a morning ritual by turning on the radio. While having it in the background, sit down and look at your vision board. Close your eyes and truly visualize what you want to achieve. Imagine walking around with your new body, feeling how healthy you are. Imagine the compliments you are receiving from all the people around you on how good you look, and imagine how comfortable you feel in your own skin. You feel lighter, fitter, agile and much more confident. While you are imagining this, try to fit this 'new you' into the picture of your goal. More specifically, think about why you are trying to achieve this and insert this 'new you' into that image. For example, if your main reason for trying to lose weight is for a specific event, imagine yourself with your new body walking into this event. Try to frame the reason in a positive light - for example, if your 'why' is that you have been told by your doctor that you must lose weight, imagine yourself being in the doctor's office as they tell you the good news about your improved bloodwork.

As you are imagining this, we need to find some way to anchor the feelings you are getting. An anchor is a psychological/physiological connection between one idea and another; this connection can be auditory, feel based, or smell. An example of an anchor is when you are out and about and you smell a perfume that reminds you of a certain person or event in your life. The connection is subconscious and you have no control over it, but just the smell of the scent can bring back very strong emotions and memories instantly. This can work equally with music, or you could attach it to a feeling.

As you get the emotions of motivation strong enough as you are visualizing, rub your thumb and forefinger together, or press them together lightly. As you do this, your subconscious is creating an association between the feelings of motivation and the finger press. At first, this will not have such a profound effect, but if you repeat this every morning it will get stronger and stronger. The higher the emotional intensity as you press your fingers together, the faster the connection will be made and the stronger it will be. That's why that perfume scent is of your first love; it was very emotional and so you will remember it forever.

You can just as effectively do this with an auditory connection. By using the function on a digital watch that creates an auditory beep every hour, we can set up a connection between the beep and the feelings of motivation. Maybe placing a photo of your watch on your vision board, or holding your watch in your hand as you go through the visualization can create a strong enough connection. The main idea is that both the feelings of motivation and the anchor you wish to connect them to are present at the same time. Now, every time your watch chimes on the hour, those motivational feelings will come flooding back to you.

This is why I asked you to put the radio on at the start of the ritual. The songs you hear at this time (when played later in the day) will subconsciously re-spark your motivation and adherence to the diet. A lot of the effectiveness of this ritual is subconscious. You may not be able to feel it working, but it will be there. Every time your watch bleeps, or every time you hear the same songs on the radio, you may get a conscious reminder to stick to your diet, along with the reasons for why you are doing so. But even if you don't, your subconscious brain is being fired in a way that will help you succeed. This works, you just need to make sure you do it.

After you have created your visualization and your anchors, read quickly through your goal sheet. This will create a further connection between the positive visuals and feelings and the goal achievement. Why not even include a phone call to the person you are being accountable to – maybe you take the time to do your workout now. Maybe you could write a small update in your blog. Whatever you include in your morning ritual, make sure it is at the start of the day as it sets up the theme for the rest of it. The whole ritual can take a minute, or much longer, depending on what you decide to include. It will, however, be the most efficient and well spent time of your life.

Overcoming Obstacles

During our journey we will come across many situations that could potentially halt or ruin our progress. In any plan, it is always worth spending some time foreseeing what could go wrong, so that we can create plans to overcome the obstacles we can face. Any business person worth his salt understands that they should go through this process so that they are fully prepared for the worst. A plan for every eventuality is a sure way to succeed in dieting, as it is in anything in life.

So what is going to stop you reaching your goal? What are potential solutions to these? Take a look at the below examples.

Problem	Solution
Meals and social events	Use calorie shuffling, meal skipping, partial fasting or full fasting to shift weekly calories around the event. Also, understanding we could also just use a maintenance calorie day to cope with this – neither a step forwards nor step back.
No motivation	Use our vision board, social accountability, re-read our goals and find out which ones fire us up the most
Negative belief	Write down as many reasons for why you deserve to be happy and achieve your goals. Look at other dramatic transformations online – see that success is possible for everyone
Making mistakes	Understand that we all make them, but have processes back in place to get back on track as soon as possible
Negative people/comments	Use it/them as fuel for motivation
Partners not helping	Make them realize you will not change as a person. Perhaps try to include them in the process somehow.

Chapter Summary

Attach your goal to a bigger reason – a why. If you can find out why you want your goal, and make that reason emotional in some way, you are more likely to achieve it.

Use both positive and negative motivational reasons. Be pulled towards something (such as more confidence) and away from other things (such as poor health).

Create a vision board – a corkboard/scrapbook/digital collage with a picture of where you are now next to pictures of where you want to be realistically.

Create a second board where you will start to put your progress pictures up next to pictures of better food choices, exercise and everything you have gained from losing weight. Make it a morning ritual to look at these boards.

Set up some form of social accountability – such as telling friends/family about your plans, blogging about it, using online forums etc.

Figure out what obstacles are going to come in your way during the process. Write down some thoughts about how you could overcome those as they pop up.

Chapter 13
Planning and Periodization

Now we enter the part where we create a plan. We have the **goal**; we know **what** we want to achieve. We also know **why** we want to achieve it, and we are focusing on that reason every day in our **morning ritual** so we have the motivation; these elements alone may be enough. Sometimes we don't need to know the 'how to' in order to be successful. Sometimes, just knowing the 'what' and the 'why' is enough to get our subconscious to find the route there. That being said, if you want to be truly successful, having a solid plan will seriously enhance your ability to achieve your goals.

In order to successfully implement the tactics in this diet, you will need to first learn them. While it is tempting to jump straight in and utilize all the ideas, it is probably a better idea to gradually employ them. For example, your first week you may want to simply cut your calories and start calorie cycling, probably the two most important aspects. When you have learned how to do this, why not start adding more lean protein to your diet. In the second month, you could even include exercising, gradually increasing in intensity as you get used to it. Potentially, should you feel up to it, try utilizing some of the fasting principles. By this point, every tactic will seem natural to you and you will be reaping the benefits.

This chapter looks at providing you with some example plans, so that you can see the diet in action and take ideas for how to implement it into your life.

Periodization and Breaks

Periodization is a more advanced planning method; it not only plans for now, but takes into account future events and how to cycle between different stages. Athletes understand periodization, as maybe they have to cycle between improving different skills/physical attributes at different times of the year. Bodybuilders go through cycles of 'bulking up' where they put on muscle and fat, followed by cycles of 'cutting', where they lose fat but try to maintain as much of the new muscle they built. Each cycle is very different and requires wholly diverse plans.

We can use the principle of periodization for ourselves in terms of creating breaks, which serve the purpose of resting, recovering and mental re-setting. Many people do not include these rests, but they are a vital component to long term success. They can not only help us break through long standing plateaus, but they can help re-ignite our motivation, and are something rewarding to look forward to. During these rest periods, we are not going to be moving forward, sometimes we may even move back slightly. But it is like the old saying, "one step back, two steps forwards". Most people take 3 steps forwards and then hit a wall, followed by slowly shuffling backwards again. We want to try to limit this.

Creating diet breaks and cycling between different periods can also decrease our risk of physical and mental burnout. Burning out is where you are trying so hard that you end up overdoing it and lose all motivation. This is often seen at the start of the year when everyone has their New Years' resolutions and are hitting the gym 5 times a week, spending 3 hours a night on the treadmill. This is simply impossible to maintain for the average person, as seen by the gym numbers slowly dwindling by the second week in January. By cycling between periods of goal achievement and rest, we are keeping motivation high (if not improving it further) and lessening our risk of injury, exhaustion and mental burnout. Everyone needs balance in their lives, and periodizing in this way can allow a well needed break that re-sets your metabolism, allowing your body to recover from the stresses of dieting. You can use these breaks as a reward for your hard work; if a break is part of the plan, you are much less likely to completely ruin your success. People who have 'accidental' breaks usually end up falling back into their old ways as they feel they have failed. This is the person who goes on holiday trying to stick to their diet, realizes they can't and so completely sabotages their goals and never gets back 'on it' again. If they had planned to allow for this scenario, it is much easier to start where they left off when the holiday has finished.

Over-motivated people struggle with this idea of periodization and including breaks. Some people think "Why should I stop now, things are going so well"? But your goals should be long term; achieving too rapidly is usually a bad sign as it can lead to all sorts of unforeseen consequences. As your results come in fast and furious, your expectations of what you can and should achieve skyrocket. This leads to feelings of despair when your results are not similar every week, thus leading to drops in motivation before falling off the bandwagon completely. Utilizing planned rest periods helps us to limit these scenarios.

Ideally, you should be in a dieting state for no longer than 3 months. As long as the diet is subtle and you take advantage of the methods in this book you should have no problem dieting for this long. Although periods longer than 3 months are easily achievable with this approach, a one week break where you eat at maintenance is recommended. Basically, during this break you will eat an amount of calories that is equivalent to your maintenance. If you have been on a diet that is in 3500 calorie weekly deficit, you would now go back to maintenance level calories (adjust this value based on your new bodyweight), depending on how your goal achievement is going. This can fire up your motivation even further, and allow your body a well deserved rest/reward. It can also boost your metabolic rate and certain hormones (such as Leptin), allowing your weight loss to be quicker when you resume the diet again. You could include these diet breaks around times that are appropriate, say if you are having a holiday or a week where you know you will be eating out a lot.

During your diet break you can also make different food choices. You can stop fasting if you were partaking in it, and you can even lower your protein intake if you wish, choosing to replace those foods with calories of your choice. Although it would be recommended to keep protein intake high if you wish to retain as much lean body mass as possible, during a maintenance week you shouldn't be losing much lean mass at all (due to the increased calories), so it shouldn't be a problem. You can continue to calorie cycle if you wish, although make the fluctuations less dramatic between your high and low days if that was the case before.

Be careful

This diet break is not an entitlement to gorge yourself silly, as you could easily put on a massive amount of weight in one week. You are still required to calorie count/be aware of calorie intake, or at the very least maintain portion control equivalent to what would maintain your weight. Remember, we are trying to ***maintain*** what we have achieved, not completely sabotage everything. You should use the diet break as information for where your metabolism currently is. If you gain too much weight during your diet break, this could be a sign that your metabolism and maintenance calories are lower than what you think. Use this as information for next time and also for when you resume your diet. You will have to change your calorie intakes as you lose weight; if you are 20 pounds lighter than when you started the diet your body will be naturally expending less calories as a result of you being smaller. So recalculate your calorie values as you progress.

It is worth mentioning that, during a maintenance week, you could easily add 2-5 pounds as a result of simply water retention. Every diet has a certain amount of bodily water loss involved with it. As a result of cycling calories and keeping carbohydrates in the diet, the fluctuation shouldn't be too great, but be aware that putting on even 5 pounds during this diet break is not as bad as you think. This weight will quickly fly off again when you resume your net cycle in the diet - so try not to worry too much if this happens.

A good way to minimize the 'shock' of water weight gain is to slowly taper off the calorie deficit as you get closer to a maintenance week. For example, during week 1-4 you may try to have a 2500 calorie weekly deficit. Through weeks 5-9 you may opt for a more aggressive 4000 calories deficit. Week 9-10 would then taper down to 2500 and then 1500 calorie deficit respectively. This would ensure that you are still losing fat weight, even as some water weight gets replaced. This tactic is highly unnecessary though. If you understand the principle of water weight fluctuations it is not a problem, as the main dilemma is purely psychological. You will not gain 5 or even 2 pounds of pure fat in a week eating at or around maintenance. It requires around 7000 - 17500 *excess* calories to do this - that is some serious overeating.

Regarding weight training, although very time efficient and effective for fat loss, it can be very demanding on the body. During the chapter on exercise, we talked about how to build up from high weights and low intensity to a more 'lean body mass sparing' regimen of lower repetitions and higher weights. This progression is important as it is necessary for your ligaments, tendons and muscles to get used to the training stress and adapt along with the gradually increasing workload. If you are to jump in and start lifting heavy straight away, you may injure yourself as your body is not ready for it yet. Utilizing rest periods, where you abstain from training, can serve an important role in allowing your body to repair, recover and move onto the next stages more efficiently. These rests should ideally coincide with your diet-breaks. Eating at maintenance calories can supply your body with the nutrients it needs for that extra recovery from the preceding weeks.

Take it easy

You could also include more frequent maintenance weeks or diet breaks if you wished. If you are 'over-achieving' (i.e. you are losing weight much faster than planned), it can be worthwhile to slow down this progress by adding an extra diet break here or there. The lessons you will learn from a diet break can be far more valuable than keeping a fast rate of weight loss going, and it will also make your weight losses much more sustainable. If you feel your motivation dwindling during the diet, you could also benefit from a diet break. Maybe you just purely cut out exercise for a week, although do not do this too frequently as exercise is an important component to your success.

Planning

So you have your goal. You have broken it down into smaller and smaller chunks until you have come to a 12-week plan. Now you need to work out what to do daily in order to achieve those goals. This simply involves breaking it down further again. Let's look at an example of a lady who would like to lose 25 pounds in a year.

25 lbs/year	=	6 lbs/12 weeks
6 lbs/12 weeks	=	½ lb/week
½ lb/week	=	~ 1750 calories deficit/week
1750 cals deficit/week	=	250 calories deficit per day

So we have taken our big yearly goal and broken it down into a daily process. We are basically trying to expend 250 calories a day more than we take in, eventually resulting in our goal. However, we must remember that weight loss is not as predictable as this, and we also are trying to allow for periodic breaks in our diet where we stay at maintenance. For these reasons, we should look to creating a bigger buffer in our plan by reaching a little higher than what we are trying to achieve. The real plan should look something more like this

40 lbs/year	=	7 ½ lbs/11 weeks (plus one week break)
7 ½ lbs/11 weeks	=	¾ pound/week
¾ pound/week	=	2800 calories deficit per week

Now we have added a buffer to our goals. By aiming for 40 pounds in a year, we should easily achieve our 25-pound goal. 40 pounds is achieved by 7 ½ pounds of weight loss every 11 weeks, plus allowance for a maintenance week. There are further buffers within the mini goals, as you will see the math does not add up perfectly for a reason. But now you have a clear idea of what you must do every week - a 2800 calorie deficit. Should you do this, you will see the weight come off and your goal should easily be met. The buffers should allow you to still achieve your goal even if things do not go exactly as planned.

The 2800 calorie deficit per week can easily be obtained by doing your exercise plan 3 times a week for half an hour at a time and a 500 calorie energy deficit in your diet on the days you are not exercising. If you have 4 days a week on dieting calories it equates to 2000 calories lost per week, easily achievable simply by skipping breakfast (if you are choosing to do intermittent fasting). The other 800 calories will come from your exercising and increase in metabolism as a result of the type of training you do.

Weekly/daily

As an example of an afternoon exerciser wishing to lose 10 pounds over 10 weeks, this person has a maintenance intake of 2300 calories per day. Their plan should look something like this;

15 pounds in 10 weeks = 1 ½ pounds per week
1 ½ pounds per week = 5500 calories per week deficit

With a plan which includes most of the elements in this book, their day would look something like this;

Time	Meal/exercise
8-12pm	Fasting
12pm-1pm	Exercise
1pm	Meal 1
5pm	Meal 2
9pm	Meal 3

They will be weight training 3 times per week, and going for a walk for half an hour twice per week. Calorie expenditure from weekly exercise would be ~ 1000 calories. Their weekly plan may look like this;

Day	Calories	Training
Mon	2000	Weights
Tues	1400	Cardio
Wed	2000	Weights
Thurs	1400	Cardio
Fri	2000	Weights
Sat	1400	Off
Sun	1400	Off

So the weekly calorie amount totals 11,600. As they need 16,100 calories to maintain their weight, this is a 4,500 calorie weekly deficit. Add on our exercise and it totals the 5,500 calorie deficit needed to lose around a pound and a half a week. If their weight loss is as predictable as this, they should lose 15 pounds over the 10 weeks. Factoring this in, it allows us to create a buffer during the 10-week plan.

Monthly

Week number	Type	Training	Predicted weight
1	Diet	Yes	-1.5 pounds
2	Diet	Yes	-3 pounds
3	Diet	Yes	-4.5 pounds
4	Diet	Yes	-6 pounds
5	Diet	Yes	-7.5 pounds
6	Maintain	No	-7.5 pounds
7	Diet	Yes	-9 pounds
8	Diet	Yes	-10.5 pounds
9	Diet	Yes	-12 pounds
10	Diet	yes	-13.5 pound
End			**-13.5 pounds**

If this person were to be losing weight faster than the 1 ½ pounds per week predicted, they may choose to include an extra diet break on week 5 or week 7. During this diet break they could also re-evaluate their goal and maybe pick a bigger one, as they are almost at their goal weight. Maybe they could just lower their weekly deficit so that the diet is a little easier and therefore more sustainable. The idea is to set your sights above what you want to achieve, but avoid achieving that higher goal too quickly. Slow down your success if you have to, which sounds counter-intuitive but makes sense when you look at long-term goals – especially with weight loss, where metabolic health is also a factor.

Assessment and Evaluation

It is hard to say which is more important - knowing why you want something, knowing how to get something or assessing whether or not you are on the right track. A goal without a 'why' is useless, that is why so many people fail with their resolutions every year. For a start, their goal is not specific enough. Add to this a lack of a reason to achieve it and you have an impotent goal. Knowing *how* to get something is equally useless if you don't have the motivation to use that knowledge. We all know those people who seem to know everything about dieting and weigh loss, yet are still out of shape themselves. But if you don't know how to get something then having the goal can sometimes be problematic. A person who really wants to lose weight but does not know how to can be left in an awful predicament. Luckily, through reading this book, you now know how to lose weight, you simply have to create the goal and the *why*. But something equally important is assessing whether or not you are on the track to your goal. If the *how* and the *why* are the bricks, the assessment is the mortar. It is the glue that holds everything in place and ensures you stay on your path. Keeping track keeps you on track.

Why assess?

There are many ways and reasons to assess yourself. You can assess yourself physically, the obvious way being to weigh yourself. However, this is my least preferred method of assessment; there are other ways that are more effective at tracking your progress. A good method or methods of assessment are very important, but the reasoning behind why you should assess yourself is even more vital.

Assessment is a great form of motivation. As you see yourself creeping towards your goal, it can inspire you immensely. The whole point of achievement is that you enjoy the process; often the goal achievement itself is not as wonderful as you would have imagined it to be. Reaching your goal can sometimes be a let-down, as the human psyche has an in built mechanism to keep striving for more; that's why even millionaires always want more money. Achieving weight loss is one of the more satisfying goals a person can strive for, but we will always find a way to make this new body of ours the 'norm' and hence it slowly loses its fulfilment-giving abilities.

By assessing correctly however, you are able to enjoy the entire process. Old clichés about "Stopping to smell the roses" and "The journey is better than the end" are very true. The process of goal achievement is an every-day event. It is an ongoing process which is constantly evolving and changing as you go through it, and through your assessment you can achieve fulfilment every step of the way. Through assessing yourself correctly, you become a scientist - every stage being a step in your development and knowledge towards understanding how *you* work and how *your* body responds. The end product is a person who is in full control of their weight and life, who has enjoyed the journey and has a new body to boot. Goals should be achieved in smaller units, every step in the process being a stride towards the ultimate goal. With each day being a small achievement in itself, it seems to snowball into an unstoppable train heading right towards the end destination.

Lack of assessment is the evil that will stop this train, and even put it into reverse. Sure, people assess their weight all the time by jumping on the scales every now and again. Putting on a pound every other week or every month or so never even registers in our minds, "maybe it's just that big meal I had last night" we tell ourselves. Within a year we have put on 10 or 12 pounds and didn't even notice it. This is not lack of assessment, but it is lack of *effective* assessment. Effective assessment is written down and evaluated, as we will find out. Left to our own devices, our mind can easily play tricks on us; it is a well known psychological tool we have developed to avoid the pain of having to deal with reality. Perhaps we even stop weighing ourselves to avoid having to face up to it; this is a very common mistake. We tell ourselves that we will just stop weighing ourselves as it is making us 'down', and that when we get ourselves and lives in order we can start again and get back into shape. Unfortunately, tomorrow never comes. However, with effective analysis of yourself, you not only boost motivation, feel more fulfilled and become more knowledgeable, but you also keep the train heading in the right direction forever.

Our analysis will be on a daily, weekly/monthly and cyclical basis. Every day you will need to focus on your process - the things you can do and control that will determine your success. This needs to be flexible enough so that, if you make a mistake one day, you can make up for it on another. Assessing results weekly can be problematic, as there can be fluctuations that affect short term figures. Assessing monthly can be more stable in terms of figures, but can limit motivation as it is too far in the future. Assessing process goals (the things you are in control of) however, can be done on a weekly and daily basis without a problem. Then we have our cycle assessment; typically 12 weeks (3 months), where we would then have a rest or maintenance week before starting our next cycle. This is a chance to compare cycles against each other, see what has improved (or hasn't in some cases) and take our learning from this to be applied to the next cycle. So let's have a look at what and how to assess effectively.

Physically

Our physical assessment will be the ultimate test of how we are doing in terms of performance. This is in our control to some level, but there are many influences outside of our control that can affect this. All we can do is take steps that give us the best chance of our physical analysis to be correct and consistent. We are going to assess three things;

Weight
Body measurements
Fat levels

Combining all of these should provide us with a very accurate view of how we are doing. Let's start with fat measurements.

I highly recommend that you get set of fat callipers. These devices are relatively cheap but can be very effective, much more so than bio impedance or fat measuring weighing scales. Even if callipers do not give you a precise measurement of your body fat percentage, you can use them to see if your measurements are heading in the right direction, as they are generally consistent from day to day. The same cannot be said of the weighing scales that claim to measure your fat percentage. If your callipers tell you that you are 20% fat, but in reality you are 25% it is not such a problem. If that number goes down, regardless of whether it is accurate or not, you will have lost fat.

To use callipers, you simply pinch some of your skin, pull it away from your body, then use the callipers to take a measurement of how thick the skin is. To make this figure more consistent, I would recommend you do it 5 times and take the middle value. Doing this at a few different sites on the body and then working out an average will give you a much more consistent value that is less susceptible to random fluctuations (such as maybe pinching a sweat gland under the skin that skews the results).

To add to this, we can use a tape measure to analyze certain parts of our body. Taking measurements for waist, hips, thighs, chest and upper arms can give us a good insight into what is happening and whether we are doing things correctly or not. Be warned, some measurements (such as waist) can fluctuate a lot based on how bloated you are, or what you have just eaten. To limit these things, measure yourself on a morning after a low calorie day. Make sure that you haven't done anything radical the night before, such as had a big meal out or a party where you drank a lot of alcohol, as these can all affect the results.

Weighing yourself is probably my least preferred method, especially short term. We have discussed how short term fluctuations in water weight can affect the results dramatically. While it is very difficult to gain 4 pounds in a week of fat mass, it is very easy to gain the same weight in water. Lots of times when we are dieting we reach a plateau. This can last 2 or even 3 weeks where we are doing everything right but weight is remaining static. Often, this is simply your body retaining water (it happens to women a lot, especially during certain times of their menstrual cycle). But fear not, just keep going with your process, and not only is your body using fat, but at some point the retained water will fly off and you will get a sudden drop in weight. Just remain patient. By utilizing your calliper and tape measurements you should be seeing some level of success here, even if your scales are being stubborn. That being said, weighing yourself is a vital component to a long term analysis plan, and should be done every 2 weeks or so. Weighing yourself once a day or once every two days in not a good idea. Not only is it nonsensical in terms of actual improvement, but it will probably drive you insane. Again, to limit any random fluctuation in water etc. try to be consistent when you weigh yourself, wearing the same clothes and making sure the previous day has been a low calorie day with nothing untoward happening the night before.

You can use these methods of analysis once every week if you wish, although it can sometimes be difficult to notice any meaningful change over this time. There are two ways around this. One is to obviously measure less frequently - once a month is not enough but once a fortnight is a nice compromise. However, you could also multiply your results by 12 or 52, to show a cycle or yearly predicted loss. For example, say you take your weekly measurement and it shows you have only lost one pound. "Great" you say, in a disheartened tone. But multiplying that by 12 equates to 12 pounds of weight loss in your 3-month cycle - not too bad. Multiply it by 52 and you have 52 pounds of loss in a year, now how do you feel about that measly pound? Doing this same tactic for fat and tape measurements could equally turn a 0.25% fat loss into a rather hefty 13% loss per year, or a 0.25 of an inch from your hips into a 3 inch loss per cycle. Why not even multiply it by 260 showing a 5 year loss (where did you disappear to?).

If you are feeling extra motivated, you could put your results into a table/chart, offering you a nice visual on your progress. This can be very rewarding to look at, as you can see your improvement very clearly. In all cases, you must write down your results and keep records of them in some way, so that you can compare from week to week, or at the very least from month to month. Do not trust yourself to keep it in your head, this consistently fails. **If the difference between your success and failure is simply writing it down**, I know what I would choose to do with those 20 seconds or so that it takes to put pen to paper. Below/next page is an example of a table you could use as a template.

Measurement	Start	Previous week	This week	Change this week
Callipers	30	25	24.5	-0.5 (6)
Hips	40	37	36.75	-0.25 (3)
Waist	35	33	33	0
Chest	40	36	35.75	-0.25 (3)
Weight	180	165	164.5	-0.5 (6)

With this table, you not only see your progress in relation to last week, but in relation to where you started, which is a good confidence boost. There are 5 main measurements, which shouldn't take long at all to obtain. Writing them down or typing the values into a spreadsheet or document will take even less time. But trust me, it is very gratifying to go through and see your successes. Your data will also provide clues as to what works best for you, helping you further in the future.

This type of physical analysis should be done for all periods of time. For example, a weekly or fortnightly one is necessary. Adding a monthly one is optional, although a 12-week cycle analysis is highly recommended. A yearly cycle analysis will help stop you 'spinning your wheels. If you are the type of person who goes on a diet for 3 months and then completely loses it ending up where you started, then this can help. Constant evaluation, even when you are not dieting, can also help to avoid this.

Mental/process evaluation

This equally important part of the diet can make or break your success. It is assessing your motivation and adherence to the diet through process means, rather than performance. This process is entirely within your control; it is the things that you do from day to day that improve your diet performance (body composition). By tracking your mental processes, you can be assured of consistent motivation and adherence to the diet. You can also spot any problems or obstacles earlier, leaping over them to get to your goal.

Put simply, you will need to analyze whether you have done what you need to on a day to day basis. The main component of your success is your calorie control, so create a table that allows you to keep track of your total calories daily. As stated before, you don't need to be precise to the nearest calorie, but try to maintain within 100-200 calorie accuracy. Placing this table with your vision board is a great way to connect the two up mentally, inspiring you to do better every day, which is what it is all about. You should put a goal amount of weekly and daily calories in the table followed with your actual calorie total taken. The result should look something like this.

Day	Goal calories	Amount eaten	Difficulty rating
Monday	1200	1300	7
Tuesday	2000	1800	2
Wednesday	1200	1400	2
Thursday	2000	2200	1
Friday	1200	1200	8
Saturday	2000	2100	3
Sunday	1200	1000	8
TOTAL	10800	11000	

With this table, we can see a goal for each day; every day is an attempt at a mini achievement. If you 'fail it' you can make up for it at some later date in the diet. A full day fast is always an option if you completely ruin your week, it could get you right back on track again (although don't do this on an exercise day). We have a weekly goal of 10800 calories, and although our example has gone over this by 200 calories they are still well under their maintenance calorie amount, so it is technically a success.

Also added to this table is a difficulty rating. This would assess on a scale of 1-10 how difficult you found the day, 10 being insanely challenging and 1 being not a problem at all. This can help you look for patterns, and can also warn you if you need a diet break. If things are getting too difficult mentally, and it is a consistent theme, maybe it is time to go on a maintenance week. Although this can slow down your short term progress, it may be better for your long term success.

Essentially, you can combine the two methods of analysis to form one sheet of analysis for both mental and physical assessment, creating one for weekly and 12-week cycle analysis. Below are some templates that you are free to copy, print and use for your own purposes.

Weekly Mental

Day	Goal calories	Amount eaten	Difficulty rating
Monday			
Tuesday			
Wednesday			
Thursday			
Friday			
Saturday			
Sunday			
TOTAL			

Physical

Measurement	Start	Last week	This week	Change this week

12 Week Cycle

Mental

Week	Goal calories	Amount eaten	Difficulty rating
1			
2			
3			
4			
5			
6			
7			
8			
9			
10			
11			
12			

Physical

Measurement	Start	Goal	End	Change this cycle

Re-evaluating

Unfortunately, we don't always achieve our goals exactly as we would like to. Life is just not as predictable as we would wish, but with persistence you will eventually get there. Sometimes we achieve our goals too quickly, this can also be a problem as it can lead to burnout. For example, if you are to lose 6 pounds in your first week it can quickly raise your expectation to the point that you anticipate this happening every week. This will lead to feelings of annoyance when this doesn't happen, and soon feelings of de-motivation will arrive. If you are doing your assessments and analysis correctly, then it should not be too much of a problem as you will see your weight loss in the bigger picture of a full cycle. Sometimes, achieving too quickly can be a sign that you have pushed yourself too hard, perhaps dropping calories too low and/or adding too much exercise. While this shows great motivation, remember it was the tortoise that won the race. For these reasons, I have outlined some strategies available to you so that you can balance out the speed of your changes.

Should our results be dramatically different to what we expected, we may have to re-evaluate our goals; maybe it needs changing, making easier or more challenging depending on what type of results you have had. Should you lose twice as much weight as planned, you may wish to 'up the ante' and try to achieve your goal in a shorter time, or strive for a bigger goal. While this is generally not my preferred suggestion, it can be a very viable option for some. On the other hand, if you have seen a lack of achievement, then you may wish to do the opposite - perhaps making an easier goal and seeing it as a more long term vision. So let's take each scenario and have a look at what we could do.

Goal missed

So you think you have been doing everything well, you have been tracking everything but nothing has changed. If it is just one week of stagnation, then it is not a problem. Continue onwards and you should see something change. Even 2 weeks of being stationary is not a problem, but if your plateau lasts 3 weeks or more then you may need to change something. Maybe the problem is you are being too one dimensional and just looking at your weight; remember that the more important statistics of body measurements and skin thickness are better indications of whether you are heading in the right direction on a week to week basis. It is not uncommon for weight to stagnate for a few weeks while we still lose fat (due to variations in body water).

The first port of call is to check whether you are being strict enough on your calorie intake or not. Are you counting those cups of coffee that have milk and sugar in them? What about that half litre of cola you had with your meal last Wednesday and Friday? Did you count the sauce on your chicken and rice? These things all add up, and while forgetting one or two things may not sabotage your success, doing it consistently will. Count everything, not obsessively to the nearest calorie, but still, count everything. Try to opt for diet soft drinks rather than the full sugar versions. Look at creating your own sauces that are low in calorie, maybe using natural flavourings such as garlic, onions, pepper, salt, vinegars, fruit juices and peels, herbs, spices, and even low fat yoghurts can be very tasty and low calorie accompaniments to a meal. Are you sticking to your daily targets? Exceeding them occasionally is not a problem, but again, consistently doing so can turn small errors into massive failures. Stop the rot before it gets too great.

If you are being very strict but you are still stagnating for a few weeks, try increasing the percentage of calories as lean protein in your diet. This is a good way of filling up for longer; 100 grams of lean meat can be as little as 100 calories. Dropping the calories on your low calorie day a little further can also help to boost the weight loss; you could even do a prolonged fast if you felt the motivation. If these two tactics fail, you could choose to drop calories on a high calorie day. While this is less optimal (it would be more preferable to have higher calories around workouts), as long as your post workout nutrition is well organized it can be a practical option. You could also choose to exercise a little longer, or add one more day to your regimen, maybe introducing cardio on your low calorie days. Try not to do more than 1 hour of exercise; this will cause you more trouble in the long run unless you have unlimited motivation.

If all of these tactics still don't kick your weight loss into action, you may have to take a maintenance week, eating slightly elevated calories so that you maintain your weight. This is a great chance to re-evaluate and re-set your goal. If you feel you are off track from your original goal and are struggling to get there, it is time to set a different goal. Extend the time period that you allow yourself to achieve that goal, and/or lower your target. For example, instead of losing 15 pounds in 10 weeks, change it to losing 10 pounds in 12 weeks. This gives you 2 more weeks to lose 5 less pounds, which is much better than quitting your goals altogether and going back to where you were. If you were listening earlier about buffers however, a small slip up can fit easily into your plan.

Over stepping your goal

While generally not seen as a problem, with our inherent human nature to always want more and more, it can quickly run us into trouble. We need to find a way to maintain a level of consistency that can be repeated almost without fail. Giant leaps, massive improvements and freak successes are rarely sustainable in the long run; more often than not they run into a brick wall. So we must take actions to slow our own success in order to keep it going for longer. The tactics presented for this are almost the opposite to the problem of missing our goal.

The first thing you should do is check your scales, make sure they are not broken. Done? Okay, now we must also put these successes into context. Did you lose 6 pounds this week with only a 2000 calories deficit? It's not fat loss for sure, maybe some water weight was shed due to a change in your diet or hormone levels. Losses of 6-10 pounds are not uncommon on a diet, especially during the start when our body rids itself of the excess food in our gut and our glycogen stores slowly deplete. Keep doing what you are doing for a few more weeks and see how it evens itself out.

If, on the other hand, you have experienced significant weight losses for a few weeks in a row, maybe it is time to re-evaluate. Any more than 3 pounds of weight loss per week and you are probably doing something wrong. Sure, it might be working, but you could also be setting yourself up for long term failure. Maybe you are losing significant amounts of lean body mass, even with the tactics we have defined to limit this negative effect of dieting. The first intervention here would be to raise calories; you are free to do this on any day you wish, low or high days is not a problem, although I would recommend placing them on days you find most difficult. Adding an extra 1500-2500 calories in a week should slow your weight loss down to a more acceptable 1-3 pounds per week.

If you are still losing weight at a rapid amount, the next idea is to cut exercise. Are you doing crazy amounts of cardio and weight training? If so, this could be going against what you want. First stage - cut out all cardio, as it is the most likely exercise to burn away your valued lean body mass. Next stage is to cut your exercise time length, making sure that you complete maybe only 2 sets of each recommended exercise per week. Keep intensity high, making sure you are lifting hard. But keep volume, or total amount of work done, to a minimum.

Maybe it is time to add in a diet and exercise break, a maintenance week. This would be a great time to catch up on some lost food, work out what your maintenance calories are and re-work your goal. If your goal was initially to lose 1 pound of steady weight per week, but you find you are losing easily 3 or more pounds, perhaps re-working your goal to a steadier 2 pound per week loss, with your ultimate goal being bigger than you initially planned. This tactic should be employed almost as a last resort after the other suggestions have been put in place.

Summary of re-evaluating

Goal not met	Goal exceeded
Continue as you are, look to your other statistics such as skin thickness	Continue as you are, seeing if it stabilizes itself
Make sure you are counting everything you eat and not missing things out, such as drinks/sauces	Increase calories on days of your choice
Increase percentage of food as protein	Cut cardio from your plan
Drop calories on low days	limit weight training to just 2 sets of each exercise per week
Drop calories on high days	Go on a maintenance week and change your goal
Increase exercise up to one hour, add some cardio	
Take a maintenance week and change your goal	

Whether you hit or miss your goal, or over exceed it in some cases, take the lessons and move on. Sometimes the lesson is that we are analysing the wrong things. Sometimes the lesson is that we hold water weight more after certain scenarios. Sometimes the lesson is to remain patient. Sometimes the lesson is to not drop our calories too much, eating closer to maintenance will allow us a slower but more consistent weight loss. Whatever it is, your analysis should help you decipher the information and take something out of it so that you can use it in your future successes.

Chapter 14

End Notes

I have used these processes in every aspect of my life, even before I turned it into such as science/method. A good example of this came for me when writing this book. I knew my goal, broke it down into smaller manageable chunks, all the way down into my daily plan. I knew my reason for wanting to create this. Helping others and sharing the knowledge that can free people from their dieting woes, essentially providing something that empowers others - this was my major motivation.

I kept a small table on my desktop assessing how many words I had written for the day. If I could just get 1,000 words a day I would have the main bulk of it completed in 2 months. By assessing this table every day, it provided the motivation to keep track and keep up with my daily targets. If I missed a day, it could be easily made up the next day or throughout the week; this is an important aspect. Initially I had a simple 'yes/no' tick box, but seeing gaps left in the table left me a little disheartened. With a small tweak, changing it to writing down how many words I had written per day, I could make up for lost ground. This made it feel more within my control, and gave me motivation to catch up with my target rather than feeling I had let myself down.

Some weeks I wrote more than my goal, some weeks less. But by constantly tweaking my goals and setting buffers, I felt as though I was progressing nicely every day. Obviously, some days I had to edit things I had written, which placed my word count to negative for the day. However, I saw this as a 'maintenance week' and continued with my process the very next day. I had to change my goal when work became busier, but by allowing myself buffers, it enabled me to hit my target in 6 months, enjoying every day the process of seeing my project create itself. Even the backward steps of editing down were seen as a forward step in the bigger picture. I used the 'breaks' to re-spark my motivation levels and create new goals, which allowed me to be supercharged when I came back to the project. Exactly how you should see your entire diet.

Maintenance of The 'New You'

This is a topic seldom talked about in diet books. Dieting is seen by most as an ongoing process, and to a certain extent it is. The people who are really successful in dieting are the ones who keep themselves there. This comes from using an approach such as the one suggested in this book; with flexibility, no restrictions on food type and psychological support, this diet is one that you can maintain for life. Other diets are death traps, as they build cravings and set up an almost guaranteed post-diet rebound of weight gain and hence depression and feelings of lack of control. This will not happen with this diet, as all of the tactics of diet breaks, analysis etc. will leave you empowered and never craving. But when you have reached your body and health goals, how should you continue?

Ideally you are not going to do much differently to what you are already doing, but just create a more user friendly diet that employs all of your favourite elements of The Flexible Diet. Continue with your physical assessments, these are vital. Without assessing yourself on a weekly or fortnightly basis, it will be very easy to slip up and start sliding backwards. Catching this before it is too late is important; it is much easier to lose that pound you accidentally gained than to go weeks without assessing and realize you have gained 10 pounds. A weekly assessment only takes 5-10 minutes (maximum) to take values and write them down, but the effects will be well worth it. We have a wonderful ability to delude ourselves into thinking we are not gaining weight; this is very quickly solved with a little analysis. Indeed, Baker and Kirschenbaum (1993) found that consistent monitoring was related to better weight loss and weight maintenance.

It would be a good idea to keep your morning ritual of looking at your success board. You don't necessarily need your vision board any longer, as you have achieved your results. Maybe you could dedicate your vision board to a new goal however. But it would be important to, at least a few times a week, have a look at the success you achieved and remind yourself of it. It can be very gratifying, and also serve as a subconscious/conscious motivator to maintain it.

You will need to work out your new caloric balance now with your lower weight. This is the best part of maintaining your new weight versus dieting down; you get to eat more food. Try not to overdo it however; we are trying to maintain, not build up again. I recommend gradually increasing the amount of calories back into your diet when you reach your goal weight. This will allow fat loss to still occur as water weight is regained, balancing itself out. But you could equally as effectively diet down to below your goal weight, so that the water weight gained from coming off the diet would take you back up to your goal weight. This is generally more psychologically difficult, as you have 'tasted' being a lower weight.

The main point of maintenance is that you will not be as obsessively counting your calories now. You do not need to keep track of calories on a daily basis, but if you like to do it then obviously you can. If you are really struggling to maintain your weight, then you may need to keep this calorie counting rule in your diet. But by being sensible about what you eat, it should not be necessary. Besides, you should have some idea of portion/calorie ratios learned by this point, so it is almost instinctive.

If you wish, continue with calorie cycling, higher levels of protein intake and fasting. If you want the health benefits associated with fasting, and/or it is just more convenient for you then do it. Fasting can allow you to experience the bigger meals without gaining weight, as long as your weekly calories are in balance. Calorie cycling will allow you to have some days of bigger meals, and higher levels of protein will be more satiating, leading to you eating generally less and feeling fuller. Try to make sure your food choices include more whole foods and micronutrient dense options, although please treat yourself occasionally too.

If you are going to stop exercising, you must account for this in your calorie intake by lowering calories until your bodyweight stabilizes. Calorie cycling and nutrient timing will become less important if you're no longer exercising. However, for maximum ability to retain what you have earned, I would strongly recommend that you continue with your exercise regimen. The suggestion I would make is to drop the volume of training by decreasing time in the gym. You should at least perform an entire body workout once a week, keeping the intensity and effort high. But you don't need to do as frequent or as long sessions, as training each body part once a week and eating at maintenance calories should ensure balance.

Try to give yourself mental boundaries and life goals. Your weight will obviously fluctuate from day to day and week to week, but by setting up limits as to what is acceptable can be very beneficial. Telling yourself that you will not go over a certain weight again, or that you will keep yourself between 'this and that' value, in weight or in measurements, can help to serve you in maintaining your weight. It is such a small thing, but to writing these boundaries down, possibly next to your success board, can help solidify them.

Maintain your physical assessments

Keep your ritual of your success board

Increase calories to maintenance

Become less obsessive about calorie counting

Decreased volume of training (if you wish)

Create acceptable boundaries

Book Summary

Educate yourself. Understand why diets work and why they fail. This can help you in your success simply through awareness.

Calorie control is king - Work out how many calories you need, and make sure you eat less than that amount with the lower limit of 1200 calories a day for women, 1600 calories a day for men (unless fasting) on average.

Cycle Calories - Alternate between one day of higher calories and one day of lower calories. You can do two high or low days in a row, but try not to stay in one condition for too long.

Protein up - Try to get between 0.8 and 1.2 grams of protein per pound of ideal bodyweight per day. Also aim to get a minimum of 25 grams of fibre a day and as many of the vitamins and minerals you need. The rest of the calories can be allocated to whatever you wish to eat.

Lift stuff - Add resistance training to your weekly routine, performing it 3 – 4 times per week for between 10 and 30 minute. If you would like, you can also add some cardio, although it is not necessary. Coincide your high calorie days with your resistance training days.

Eat what you like – with The Flexible Diet, you don't have to cut out any foods. You can still eat all the foods you love, just make sure the rules of the diet are adhered to (particularly calorie control). Also, try to include as much nutrient-dense and calorie-light foods, such as fruits and vegetables.

Eat when you like – prefer big breakfasts? Late night feasts? Go ahead, eat when you want. You can even skip a meal if you like and eat a bit more later in the day, or vice versa. As long as the other rules of the diet are adhered to, feel free to choose your own meal frequency and timing. Although try to get adequate post workout nutrition in the 24 hours after your workout.

Don't eat sometimes – try fasting if you want to gain some of the health benefits and potential weight management benefits. Ease yourself into it by perhaps doing a 16 hour fast (skip breakfast), before attempting to extend all the way to a full day fast. Alternatively, you could do intermittent fasting daily.

Get Clear – write out your goals. Find out what your motivation is for achieving weight loss and focus on this. Set out a solid plan and evaluate it regularly.

Assess yourself – use weighing scales, measuring tape and callipers, as well as monitoring daily and weekly calories. See if you are heading in the right direction.

Re-assess – we need to be flexible in our approach, so you need to occasionally re-assess your goals and change them as you see fit. Never give up – just change the pace.

Take a break - Set out diet breaks so that you have a resting point to reach before continuing your journey.

Maintain - Enjoy the 'new you' and your new found control over your diet, your weight, your happiness and your life. Maintenance of a stable weight is just as important as getting there – if not more.

Good luck in your Journey

References

Adlouni A, Ghalim N, Benslimane A, Lecerf JM, Saile R. (1997). Fasting during Ramadan induces a marked increase in high density lipoprotein cholesterol and decrease in low-density lipoprotein cholesterol. *Ann. Nutr. Metab.* 41:242–49

Ahmed T, Sai Krupa Das, Julie K. Golden, Edward Saltzman, Susan B. Roberts, and Simin Nikbin Meydani. (2009). Calorie Restriction Enhances T-Cell–Mediated Immune Response in Adult Overweight Men and Women. *J Gerontol A Biol Sci Med Sci* 64A (11): 1107-1113

Anson RM, Guo Z, de Cabo R, Iyun T, Rios M, Hagepanos A, Ingram DK, Lane MA, Mattson MP. Intermittent fasting dissociates beneficial effects of dietary restriction on glucose metabolism and neuronal resistance to injury from calorie intake. Proc Natl Acad Sci U S A. 2003 May 13;100(10):6216-20.

Aragon, A.A. and Schoenfeld, B.J. (2013) Nutrient timing revisited: is there a post-exercise anabolic window? Journal of the International Society of Sports Nutrition 2013, 10:5 doi:10.1186/1550-2783-10-5

Arnal MA, et al. Protein feeding pattern does not affect protein retention in young women. J Nutr. 2000 Jul;130(7):1700-4.

Andersen LL, Tufekovic G, Zebis MK, et al. The effect of resistance training combined with timed ingestion of protein on muscle fiber size and muscle strength. Metabolism. Feb 2005;54(2):151 – 156.

Aston LM1, Stokes CS, Jebb SA.(2008) No effect of a diet with a reduced glycaemic index on satiety, energy intake and body weight in overweight and obese women. Int J Obes (Lond). 2008 Jan;32(1):160-5. Epub 2007 Oct 9.

Baker R. C, and Kirschenbaum, D. S. (1993) Self-monitoring may be necessary for successful weight control. Journal of Behavior therapy 24, 377-394

Bellisle F, McDevitt R, Prentice AM. (1997). Meal frequency and energy balance. Br J Nutr. 77 Suppl 1:S57-70.

Bhutani S, Klempel MC, Berger RA, Varady KA. Improvements in Coronary Heart Disease Risk Indicators by Alternate-Day Fasting Involve Adipose Tissue Modulations. Obesity (Silver Spring). 2010 Mar 18.

Gianni, B. Tipton, KD. Klein, S. and Wolfe, RR. An abundant supply of amino acids enhances the metabolic effect of exercise on muscle protein. Am. J. Physiol. 273 (Endocrinol. Metab. 36): E122-E129, 1997.

Blumenthal JA; Babyak, MA; Sherwood, A; Craighead, L; Lin, P; Johnson, J; Watkins, LL; Wang, JT; Kuhn, C; Feinglos, M; Hinderliter, A. (2010). Effects of the Dietary Approaches to Stop Hypertension Diet Alone and in Combination With Exercise and Caloric Restriction on Insulin Sensitivity and Lipids *Hypertension* ;55;1199-1205

Cameron JD, Cyr MJ, Doucet E. (2010). Increased meal frequency does not promote greater weight loss in subjects who were prescribed an 8 week equi-energetic energy restricted diet. *Br J Nutr*. 103(8):1098-101

Burke LM, Collier GR, Hargreaves M. Muscle glycogen storage after prolonged exercise: effect of the glycemic index of carbohydrate feedings. J Appl Physiol. (1993) Aug;75(2):1019-23.

Carlson, Anton J. and Frederick Hoelzel. Apparent Prolongation of the Life Span of Rats by Intermittent Fasting. Journal of Nutrition Vol. 31 No. 3 March 1946, pp. 363-375

Chaston TB, Dixon JB, O'Brien PE. Changes in fat-free mass during significant weight loss: a systematic review. Int J Obes (Lond). 2007 May;31(5):743-50. Epub 2006 Oct 31.

Cho S, Dietrich M, Brown CJ, Clark CA, Block G. (2003). The effect of breakfast type on total daily energy intake and body mass index: results from the Third National Health and Nutrition Examination Survey.. *J am Coll Nut.* Aug;22(4):296-302.

Chomentowski P, John J. Dubé, Francesca Amati, Maja Stefanovic-Racic, Shanjian Zhu, Frederico G.S. Toledo and Bret H. Goodpaster. (2009). Moderate Exercise Attenuates the Loss of Skeletal Muscle Mass That Occurs With Intentional Caloric Restriction–Induced Weight Loss in Older, Overweight to Obese Adults. *J Gerontol A Biol Sci Med Sci.* 64A (5): 575-580. doi: 10.1093

Cribb, PJ; Hayes, A. (2006). Effects of Supplement Timing and Resistance Exercise on Skeletal Muscle Hypertrophy Medicine & Science in Sports & Exercise: November 2006 - Volume 38 - Issue 11 - pp 1918-1925

Das SK, Gilhooly CH, Golden JK, Pittas AG, Fuss PJ, Cheatham RA, Tyler S, Tsay M, McCrory MA, Lichtenstein AH, Dallal GE, Dutta C, Bhapkar MV, Delany JP, Saltzman E, Roberts SB. Long-term effects of 2 energy-restricted diets differing in glycemic load on dietary adherence, body composition, and metabolism in CALERIE: a 1-y randomized controlled trial. Am J Clin Nutr. 2007 Apr;85(4):1023-30.

Dansinger ML, Gleason JA, Griffith JL, Selker HP, Schaefer EJ. (2005). Comparison of the Atkins, Ornish, Weight Watchers, and Zone diets for weight loss and heart disease risk reduction: a randomized trial. *JAMA.*;293(1):43-53.

Descamps O, Riondel J, Ducros V, Roussel AM. Mitochondrial production of reactive oxygen species and incidence of age-associated lymphoma in OF1 mice: effect of alternate-day fasting. Mech Ageing Dev (2005);126:1185–91

Deutz, Nicolaas EP and Wolfe, Robert R (2013) Is there a maximal anabolic response to protein intake with a meal? Clin Nutr. 2013 Apr; 32(2): 309–313.

Duan, W.; Guo, Z; Jiang, H; Ware, M; Li, XJ; Mattson, MP (2003). "Dietary restriction normalizes glucose metabolism and BDNF levels, slows disease progression, and increases survival in huntingtin mutant mice". Proceedings of the National Academy of Sciences 100 (5): 2911–6

Dube' JJ, Francesca Amati, Maja Stefanovic-Racic, Frederico G. S. Toledo, Sarah E. Sauers, and Bret H. Goodpaster. (2008). Exercise-induced alterations in intramyocellular lipids and insulin resistance:the athlete's paradox revisited. *Am J Physiol Endocrinol Metab* 294: E882–E888,

Eshghinia and Mohammadzadeh (2013). The effects of modified alternate-day fasting diet on weight loss and CAD risk factors in overweight and obese women. Journal of Diabetes & Metabolic Disorders 2013, 12:4

Esmarck B, J L Andersen, S Olsen, E A Richter, M Mizuno and M Kjær. (2001). Timing of postexercise protein intake is important for muscle hypertrophy with resistance training in elderly humans. The Journal of Physiology, *535,* 301-311.

Fatouros IG, Chatzinikolaou A, Tournis S, Nikolaidis MG, Jamurtas AZ, Douroudos II, Papassotiriou I, Thomakos PM, Taxildaris K, Mastorakos G, Mitrakou A. (2009). Intensity of resistance exercise determines adipokine and resting energy expenditure responses in overweight elderly individuals. Diabetes Care. 32(12):2161-7

Flakoll PJ, Judy T, Flinn K, Carr C, Flinn S. (2004) Postexercise protein supplementation improves health and muscle soreness during basic military training in marine recruits. J Appl Physiol. Mar 2004;96(3):951 – 956.

Fontana L, Timothy E. Meyer , Samuel Klein, and John O. Holloszy. (2004). Long-term calorie restriction is highly effective in reducing the risk for atherosclerosis in humans. *PNAS*. **vol. 101 no. 17** 6659-6663

Garthe I[1], Raastad T, Refsnes PE, Koivisto A, Sundgot-Borgen J. (2011). Effect of two different weight-loss rates on body composition and strength and power-related performance in elite athletes. Int J Sport Nutr Exerc Metab. 2011 Apr;21(2):97-104

Goodpaster BH, PhD, James P. DeLany, PhD, Amy D. Otto, PhD, Lewis Kuller, MD, Jerry Vockley, MD, PhD, Jeannette E. South-Paul, MD, Stephen B. Thomas, PhD, Jolene Brown, MD, Kathleen McTigue, MD, MS, MPH, Kazanna C. Hames, MS,Wei Lang, PhD, John M. Jakicic, PhD (2010). Effects ofDiet and Physical Activity Interventions onWeight Loss and Cardiometabolic Risk Factors in Severely Obese Adults *JAMA,*—Vol 304, No. 16

Goodpaster BH, Kelley DE, Wing RR, Meier A, Thaete FL. (1999). Effects of weight loss on regional fat distribution and insulin sensitivity in obesity. *Diabetes*;48:839–47

P. L. Greenhaff, L. G. Karagounis, N. Peirce, E. J. Simpson, M. Hazell, R. Layfield, H. Wackerhage, K. Smith, P. Atherton, A. Selby, and M. J. Rennie (2008). Disassociation between the effects of amino acids and insulin on signaling, ubiquitin ligases, and protein turnover in human muscle AJP - Endo **September 2008 vol. 295 no. 3** E595-E604

Halagappa VK, Guo Z, Pearson M, Matsuoka Y, Cutler RG, Laferla FM, Mattson MP. (2007) Intermittent fasting and caloric restriction ameliorate age-related behavioral deficits in the triple-transgenic mouse model of Alzheimer's disease. Neurobiol Dis. 2007 Apr;26(1):212-20.

Halberg Nils, Morten Henriksen, Nathalie Söderhamn, Bente Stallknecht, Thorkil Ploug, PeterSchjerling, Flemming Dela. Journal of Applied Physiology Published 1 December (2005) Vol. 99 no. 6, 2128-2136 DOI: 10.1152/japplphysiol.00683.2005

Harvie N M, M Pegington, M P Mattson, J Frystyk, B Dillon, G Evans, J Cuzick, S A Jebb, B Martin, R G Cutler, T G Son, S Maudsley, O D Carlson, J M Egan, A Flyvbjerg and A Howell1 The effects of intermittent or continuous energy restriction on weight loss and metabolic disease risk markers: a randomized trial in young overweight women International Journal of Obesity (2011) 35, 714–727; doi:10.1038/ijo.2010.171

Heden T, Lox C, Rose P, Reid S, Kirk EP. (2011). One-set resistance training elevates energy expenditure for 72 h similar to three sets. Eur J Appl Physiol.(3):477-84.

Heilbronn LK, Smith SR, Martin CK, Anton S, Ravussin E. (2005). Alternate day fasting in nonobese subjects: effects on body weight, body composition, and energy metabolism. *Am. J. Clin. Nutr.* 81:69–73

Heilbronn, LK PhD; Lilian de Jonge, PhD; Madlyn I. Frisard, PhD; James P. DeLany, PhD; D. Enette Larson-Meyer, PhD; Jennifer Rood, PhD; Tuong Nguyen, BSE; Corby K. Martin, PhD; Julia Volaufova, PhD; Marlene M. Most, PhD; Frank L. Greenway, PhD; Steven R. Smith, MD; Walter A. Deutsch, PhD; Donald A. Williamson, PhD; Eric Ravussin, PhD; (2006). Effect of 6-Month Calorie Restriction on Biomarkers of Longevity, Metabolic Adaptation, and Oxidative Stress in Overweight Individuals *JAMA.*;**295(13)**:1539-1548

Hendler, R.G, Walesky, M, Sherwin, R (1985) Sucrose substitution in prevention and reversal of the fall in metabolic rate accompanying hypocaloric diets. The American Journal of Medicine Volume 81, Issue 2 , 280-284

Holmstrup ME, Christopher M. Owens, Timothy J. Fairchild, Jill A. Kanaley (2010). Effect of meal frequency on glucose and insulin excursions over the course of a day. The European e-Journal of Clinical Nutrition and Metabolism 5 (2010) e277ee280

Holt SHA, Miller J CB and Petocz P (1997). An insulin index of foods: the insulin demand generated by 1000kj portions of common foods, American journal of clinical nutrition, vol66 no. 5

Honjoh S, Yamamoto T, Uno M, Nishida E. (2008). Signalling through RHEB-1 mediates intermittent fasting-induced longevity in C. elegans. Nature.

Houmard JA, Charles J. Tanner, Chunli Yu, Paul G. Cunningham, Walter J. Pories, Kenneth G. MacDonald and Gerald I. Shulman. (2002). Effect of Weight Loss on Insulin Sensitivity and Intramuscular Long-Chain Fatty Acyl-CoAs in Morbidly Obese Subjects. *Diabetes*. **vol. 51 no. 10** 2959-2963

Hsieh EA, Chai CM, Hellerstein MK. (2005). Effects of caloric restriction on cell proliferation in several tissues in mice: role of intermittent feeding. Am J Physiol Endocrinol Metab 2005;288

Hu T1, Mills KT, Yao L, Demanelis K, Eloustaz M, Yancy WS Jr, Kelly TN, He J, Bazzano LA. (2012). Effects of low-carbohydrate diets versus low-fat diets on metabolic risk factors: a meta-analysis of randomized controlled clinical trials. Am J Epidemiol. 2012 Oct 1;176 Suppl 7:S44-54. doi: 10.1093/aje/kws264.

http://intermountainhealthcare.org/hospitals/imed/about/news/Pages/home.aspx?NewsID=713

Ivy JL, Katz AL, Cutler CL, Sherman WM, Coyle EF, Muscle glycogen synthesis after exercise: effect of time of carbohydrate ingestion, J Appl Physiol. 1988 Apr;64(4):1480-5.

Johnson, J; Laub, D; John, S (2006). "The effect on health of alternate day calorie restriction: Eating less and more than needed on alternate days prolongs life". Medical Hypotheses 67 (2): 209–11

Johnson JB, Summer W, Cutler RG, Martin B, Hyun DH, Dixit VD, Pearson M, Nassar M, Telljohann R, Maudsley S, Carlson O, John S, Laub DR, Mattson MP. (2007). Alternate day calorie restriction improves clinical findings and reduces markers of oxidative stress and inflammation in overweight adults with moderate asthma. Free Radic Biol Med;43(9):1348

Johnson, James B.; Summer, Warren; Cutler, Roy G.; Martin, Bronwen; Hyun, Dong-Hoon; Dixit, Vishwa D.; Pearson, Michelle; Nassar, Matthew et al. (2007). "Alternate Day Calorie Restriction Improves Clinical Findings and Reduces Markers of Oxidative Stress and Inflammation in Overweight Adults with Moderate Asthma". Free Radical Biology and Medicine 42 (5): 665–74

Johnston CS, Sherrie L Tjonn, Pamela D Swan, Andrea White, Heather Hutchins, and Barry Sears. (2006). Ketogenic low-carbohydrate diets have no metabolic advantage over nonketogenic low-carbohydrate diets. Am J Clin Nutr;83:1055–61.

Johnstone AM, Stubbs RJ, Harbron CG. (1996). Effect of overfeeding macronutrients on day-to-day food intake in man. Eur J Clin Nutr.(7):418-30.

Katare RG, Kakinuma Y, Arikawa M, Yamasaki F, Sato T. (2009). Chronic intermittent fasting improves the survival following large myocardial ischemia by activation of BDNF/VEGF/PI3K signaling pathway. J Mol Cell Cardiol. 2009 Mar;46(3):405-12.

Kessler D (2009) the end of overeating

Keim NL, Van Loan MD, Horn WF, Barbieri TF, Mayclin PL.(1997). Weight loss is greater with consumption of large morning meals and fat-free mass is preserved with large evening meals in women on a controlled weight reduction regimen. J Nutr. 1997 Jan; 127(1): 75-82.

Kirk EP, Donnelly JE, Smith BK, Honas J, Lecheminant JD, Bailey BW, Jacobsen DJ, Washburn RA. (2009). Minimal resistance training improves daily energy expenditure and fat oxidation. Med Sci Sports Exerc. 41(5):1122-9.

René Koopman, Anton J. M. Wagenmakers, Ralph J. F. Manders, Antoine H. G. Zorenc, Joan M. G. Senden, Marchel Gorselink, Hans A. Keizer, and Luc J. C. van Loon. (2005). Combined ingestion of protein and free leucine with carbohydrate increases postexercise muscle protein synthesis in vivo in male subjects. 2005 vol. 288 no. 4 E645-E653 American Journal of Physiology

Kreitzman S N, Coxon A Y, and Szaz K F. (1992) storage: illusions of easy weight loss, excessive weight regain, and distortions in estimates of body composition. The American Society for Clinical Nutrition Glycogen

Lane MA, Baer DJ, Rumpler WV, Weindruch R, Ingram DK, Tilmont EM, Cutler RG, Roth GS. (1996). Calorie restriction lowers body temperature in rhesus monkeys, consistent with a postulated anti-aging mechanism in rodents. Proc Natl Acad Sci U S A. 1996 Apr 30;93(9):4159-64.

La Bounty PM, Bill I Campbell, Jacob Wilson, Elfego Galvan, John Berard, Susan M Kleiner, Richard B Kreider, Jeffrey R Stout, Tim Ziegenfuss, Marie Spano, Abbie Smith, Jose Antonio (2011) International Society of Sports Nutrition position stand: meal frequency. Journal of the International Society of Sports Nutrition, 8:4

Leidy HJ, Clifton PM, Astrup A, Wycherley TP, Westerterp-Plantenga MS, Luscombe-Marsh ND, Woods SC, Mattes RD. (2015). The role of protein in weight loss and maintenance. Am J Clin Nutr. 2015 Apr 29. pii: ajcn084038.

Levenhagen, D. K., C. Carr, M. G. Carlson, D. J. Maron, M. J. Borel, and P. J. Flakoll. (2002). Postexercise protein intake enhances whole-body and leg protein accretion in humans. *Med. Sci. Sports Exerc.*, Vol. 34, No. 5, pp. 828-837, 2002.

Lim EL[1], Hollingsworth KG, Aribisala BS, Chen MJ, Mathers JC, Taylor R. (2011). Reversal of type 2 diabetes: normalisation of beta cell function in association with decreased pancreas and liver triacylglycerol. Diabetologia. 2011 Oct;54(10):2506-14. doi: 10.1007/s00125-011-2204-7. Epub 2011 Jun 9.

Mansell PI, Fellows IW, Macdonald IA. (1990). Enhanced thermogenic response to epinephrine after 48-h starvation in humans. *Am J Physiol.* Jan;258(1 Pt 2):R87-93

Martin A, Normand S, Sothier M, Peyrat J, Louche-Pelissier C, Laville M. (2000). Is advice for breakfast consumption justified? Results from a short-term dietary and metabolic experiment in young healthy men. *Br. J. Nutr.* 84:337–44

Mattson MP. (2000). Neuroprotective signaling and the aging brain: take away my food and let me run. Brain Res. Dec 15;886(1-2):47-53.

Mark P. Mattson. (2005). Energy Intake, Meal Frequency and Health: A Neurobiological Perspective* Annual Review of Nutrition Vol. 25: 237-260

Meyer TE PhD, Sándor J. Kovács PhD, MD, Ali A. Ehsani MD, Samuel Klein MD, John O. Holloszy MD and Luigi Fontana MD, PhD. (2006). Long-Term Caloric Restriction Ameliorates the

Decline in Diastolic Function in Humans. Journal of the American College of Cardiology. Volume 47, Issue 2, Pages 398-402

Miller SL, Tipton KD, Chinkes DL, Wolf SE, Wolfe RRIndependent and combined effects of amino acids and glucose after resistance exercise. Med Sci Sports Exerc. 2003 Mar;35(3):449-55.

Moran LJ, Luscombe-Marsh ND, Noakes M, Wittert GA, Keogh JB, Clifton PM.(2005). The satiating effect of dietary protein is unrelated to postprandial ghrelin secretion. J Clin Endocrinol Metab. 90(9):5205-11

Nicklas TA, Morales M, Linares A, Yang SJ, Baranowski T, et al. (2004). Children's meal patterns have changed over a 21-year period: the Bogalusa Heart Study. *J. Am. Diet. Assoc.* 104:753–61

Nils Halberg, Morten Henriksen, Nathalie Söderhamn, Bente Stallknecht, Thorkil Ploug, Peter Schjerling, and Flemming Dela. (2005). Effect of intermittent fasting and refeeding on insulin action in healthy men Journal of Applied Physiology. **vol. 99no. 6** 2128-2136

Noakes M, Keogh JB, Foster PR, Clifton PM. (2005). Effect of an energy-restricted, high-protein, low-fat diet relative to a conventional high-carbohydrate, low-fat diet on weight loss, body composition, nutritional status, and markers of cardiovascular health in obese women. The American Journal of Clinical Nutrition, 81(6):1298-1306]

Noakes M, et al. (2006) Comparison of isocaloric very low carbohydrate/high saturated fat and high carbohydrate/low saturated fat diets on body composition and cardiovascular risk. Nutr Metab (Lond). 11;3:7.

O'Leary VB, Marchetti CM, Krishnan RK, Stetzer BP, Gonzalez F, Kirwan JP. (2006) Exercise-induced reversal of insulin resistance in obese elderly is associated with reduced visceral fat. J Appl Physiol. 100(5):1584-9.

Paddon-Jones D, Westman E, Mattes RD, Wolfe RR, Astrup A, Westerterp-Plantenga M.(2008). Protein, weight management, and satiety. Am J Clin Nutr. 87(5):1558S-1561S.

Park, Yikyung Sc.D; Subar, Amy F Ph.D; Hollenbeck, Albert Ph.D; and Schatzkin, Arthur MD (2011). Dietary fiber intake and mortality in the NIH-AARP Diet and Health Study Arch Intern Med; 171(12): 1061–1068.

Porrata Carmen, MD, PhD, Julio Sánchez, MD, Violeta Correa, MD, Alfredo Abuín, MD, Manuel Hernández-Triana, MD, PhD, Raúl Vilá Dacosta-Calheiros, MD, María Elena Díaz, PhD, Mayelín Mirabal, MS, Eduardo Cabrera, PhD, Concepción Campa, MS, Mario Pianesi. (2009). Ma-Pi 2 Macrobiotic Diet Intervention in Adults with Type 2 Diabetes Mellitus MEDICC Review » Fall 2009, Vol 11, No 4

Romon M, Lebel P, Velly C, Marecaux N, Fruchart JC, Dallongeville J. (1999). Leptin response to carbohydrate or fat meal and association with subsequent satiety and energy intake. Am J Physiol. 1999 Nov;277(5 Pt 1):

Roth GS, Lane MA, Ingram DK, et al. (2002). Biomarkers of caloric restriction may predict longevity in humans. Science;297:811

Ryan AS. (2000). Insulin resistance with aging: effects of diet and exercise. Sports Med. Nov;30(5):327-46.

Siegel I, Liu TL, Nepomuceno N, Gleicher N. (1988). Effects of short-term dietary restriction on survival of mammary ascites tumor-bearing rats. Cancer Invest;6:677–80

Smith CF, Williamson DA, Bray GA, Ryan DH. (1999). Flexible vs. Rigid dieting strategies: relationship with adverse behavioral outcomes. Appetite. 1999 Jun;32(3):295-305.

Soare Andreea, Yeganeh M Khazrai, Rossella Del Toro, Elena Roncella, Lucia Fontana, Sara Fallucca, Silvia Angeletti, Valeria Formisano, Francesca Capata, Vladimir Ruiz, Carmen Porrata, Edlira Skrami, Rosaria Gesuita, Silvia Manfrini, Francesco Fallucca, Mario Pianesi, and Paolo Pozzilli. (2014). The effect of the macrobiotic Ma-Pi 2 diet vs. the recommended diet in the management of type 2 diabetes: the randomized controlled MADIAB trial Nutrition & Metabolism, 11:39

Soeters MR, et al. (2009). Intermittent fasting does not affect whole-body glucose, lipid, or protein metabolism. Am J Clin Nutr;90(5):1244-51.

Solomon TP, Sistrun SN, Krishnan RK, Del Aguila LF, Marchetti CM, O'Carroll SM, O'Leary VB, Kirwan JP. (2008) Exercise and diet enhance fat oxidation and reduce insulin resistance in older obese adults. J Appl Physiol. 104(5):1313-9.

Soenen S, Bonomi AG, Lemmens SG, Scholte J, Thijssen MA, van Berkum F, Westerterp-Plantenga MS. (2012). Relatively high-protein or 'low-carb' energy-restricted diets for body weight loss and body weight maintenance? Physiol Behav. 2012 Oct 10;107(3):374-80. doi: 10.1016/j.physbeh.2012.08.004.

Sofer S, Eliraz A, Kaplan S, Voet H, Fink G, Kima T, Madar Z. Greater weight loss and hormonal changes after 6 months diet with carbohydrates eaten mostly at dinner. (2011). Obesity (Silver Spring);19(10):2006-14.

Stephens BR, Sautter JM, Holtz KA, Sharoff CG, Chipkin SR, Braun B. (2007). Effect of timing of energy and carbohydrate replacement on post-exercise insulin action. Appl Physiol Nutr Metab.;32(6):1139-47.

Stewart W.K and Laura W. Fleming. (1973). Features of a successful therapeutic fast of 382 days' duration Postgrad Med J49(569): 203–209.

Stewart TM1, Williamson DA, White MA. (2002). Rigid vs. flexible dieting: association with eating disorder symptoms in nonobese women. Appetite. 2002 Feb;38(1):39-44.

Stote KS1, Baer DJ, Spears K, Paul DR, Harris GK, Rumpler WV, Strycula P, Najjar SS, Ferrucci L, Ingram DK, Longo DL, Mattson MP. (2007) A controlled trial of reduced meal frequency without caloric restriction in healthy, normal-weight, middle-aged adults. Am J Clin Nutr. Apr;85(4):981-8.

Surwit RS, Feinglos MN, McCaskill CC, Clay SL, Babyak MA, Brownlow BS, Plaisted CS, Lin PH. (1997). Metabolic and behavioral effects of a high-sucrose diet during weight loss. Am J Clin Nutr. Apr;65(4):908-15.

Swinburn B, Gary Sacks, and Eric Ravussin. (2009). Increased food energy supply is more than sufficient to explain the US epidemic of obesity. Am J Clin Nutr. vol. 90 no. 6 **1453-1456**

Tang, J.E et al. (2007). Minimal whey protein with carbohydrate stimulates muscle protein synthesis following resistance exercise in trained young men. Appl Phisiol Nutr metab. 32 (6); 1132-1138

Teixeira PJ, Scott B. Going, Linda B. Houtkooper, Lauve L. Metcalfe, Robert M. Blew, Hilary G. Flint-Wagner, Ellen C. Cussler, Luís B. Sardinha, and Timothy G.Lohman. (2003). Resistance training in postmenopausal women with and without hormone therapy. Med Sci Sports Exerc;35(4):555-62.

Tipton KD, Arny A. Ferrando, Stuart M. Phillips, David Doyle Jr., Robert R. Wolfe. (1999). Postexercise net protein synthesis in human muscle from orally administered amino acids. Am J Physiol Endocrinol Metab 276:E628-E634.

Varady KA, Surabhi Bhutani, Emily C Church, and Monica C Klempel. (2009). Short-term modified alternate-day fasting: a novel dietary strategy forweight loss and cardioprotection in obese adults. Am J Clin Nutr 90:1138–43

Varady KA. (2011). Intermittent versus daily calorie restriction: which diet regimen is more effective for weight loss? Obes Rev. Jul;12(7)

Wingard DL, Berkman LF, Brand RJ. (1982). A multivariate analysis of health related practices: a nine-year mortality follow-up of the Alameda County Study. *Am. J. Epidemiol.* 116:765–75

Weigle DS, Breen PA, Matthys CC, Callahan HS, Meeuws KE, Burden VR, Purnell JQ. (2005). A high-protein diet induces sustained reductions in appetite, ad libitum caloric intake, and body weight despite compensatory changes in diurnal plasma Leptin and ghrelin concentrations. Am J Clin Nutr. 2005 Jul;82(1):41-8.

Westerterp-Plantenga MS. (2003). The significance of protein in food intake and body weight regulation. Curr Opin Clin Nutr Metab Care.;6(6):635-8.

Willoughby DS, Stout JR, Wilborn CD. (2006). Effects of resistance training and protein plus amino acid supplementation on muscle anabolism, mass, and strength. Amino Acids.

Wu B-H, Jung-Charng Lin. (2006.) Effects of Exercise Intensity on Excess Post-Exercise Oxygen Consumption and Substrate use After Resistance Exercise. J Exerc Sci Fit , Vol 4, No 2,

Yukiko N; Oshima, Tetsuya; Sasaki, Shota; Higashi, Yukihito; Ozono, Ryoji; Takenaka, Sou; Miura, Fumiharu; Hirao, Hidekazu; Matsuura, Hideo; Chayama, Kazuaki; Kambe, Masayuki.

(2001). Calorie Restriction Reduced Blood Pressure in Obesity Hypertensives by Improvement of Autonomic Nerve Activity and Insulin Sensitivity. Journal of Cardiovascular Pharmacology: Volume 38 - Issue - p S69–S74

Zauner C, Bruno Schneeweiss, Alexander Kranz, Christian Madl, Klaus Ratheiser, Ludwig Kramer, Erich Roth, Barbara Schneider, and Kurt Lenz. (2000). Resting energy expenditure in short-term starvation is increased as a result of an increase in serum norepinephrine. Am J Clin Nutr. **vol. 71** *no. 6* 1511-1515

Made in the USA
Middletown, DE
29 September 2018